Monika Gupta
Anshuman Jamdade
Amrita Aggarwal

A VISUAL SYMPHONY OF SALIVARY GLAND IMAGING

Monika Gupta
Anshuman Jamdade
Amrita Aggarwal

A VISUAL SYMPHONY OF SALIVARY GLAND IMAGING

A Diagnostic Journey Through Salivary Gland Structure and Disease, Revealed Through Advanced Imaging

LAP LAMBERT Academic Publishing

Imprint

Cover image: www.ingimage.com

Publisher:
LAP LAMBERT Academic Publishing
is a trademark of
Dodo Books Indian Ocean Ltd. and OmniScriptum S.R.L publishing group

120 High Road, East Finchley, London, N2 9ED, United Kingdom
Str. Armeneasca 28/1, office 1, Chisinau MD-2012, Republic of Moldova, Europe
Managing Directors: Ieva Konstantinova, Victoria Ursu
info@omniscriptum.com

Printed at: see last page
ISBN: 978-620-8-44245-3

A VISUAL SYMPHONY OF SALIVARY GLAND IMAGING

Author

Dr. Monika Gupta

Co-Author

Dr. Anshuman Jamdade (BDS, MDS)
Professor & Head of Department
Oral Medicine & Radiology

Dr. Satyapal Yadav (BDS, MDS)
Professor
Oral Medicine & Radiology

Dr.Neeraj Kumar (BDS, MDS)
Professor
Oral Medicine & Radiology

Dr. Amrita Aggarwal (BDS, MDS)
Reader
Oral Medicine & Radiology

ACKNOWLEDGEMENT

This Research work was possible only because of great efforts put by large number of people. It would leave a void in this dissertation, if their efforts are not acknowledged.

First of all, I would like to thank the Almighty god for giving me a good life.
I am eternally obliged to lot of kind individuals who have helped me whole heartedly during every step of this research work and have reaffirmed my faith in human nature. I am very grateful to my grandparents **Late Sh. Ramlal Gupta and Late Smt. Leela devi Gupta** for their unconditional love and blessings, my parents **Mr. Navratan Gupta & Mrs. Kamlesh Gupta**, for their patience and support and making me what I am today. Without their support, I would not be able to purse my post-graduation. At the very onset I would like to convey my heartful gratitude to my parents who have been the backbone in every aspect of my life.

I am highly obliged for the extensive guidance and assistance rendered to me by my guide **Dr. Anshuman Jamdade**, Professor and Head of Department of Oral Medicine & Radiology, Mahatma Gandhi Dental College and Hospital, Jaipur. His patience and support helped me to complete this research work under his guidance in the most beautiful manner it could have been. I am fortunate to be under his unlimited source of knowledge, skill and the perfection he desires in his work and sees in his students.

I express my deepest gratitude to **Dr. Satyapal Yadav** (Professor & Co Guide), **Dr.Neeraj Yadav** (Professor), **Dr. Amrita Aggarwal** (Reader) for their expert opinion, motivation and support during the preparation of this study and throughout my post graduate course.
I would like to post my sincere thanks to my colleague **Dr Kanishka Singh**, **Dr Saurabh Kanawa** for being a greatest support & helping hand throughout. I immensely thanks to my seniors **Dr Anuja Sharma** and **Dr Kanupriya Sharma** and my junior **Dr Reeya Garg** for their constant care, support and stood by me whenever I needed them the most.

I would like to post my heartful thanks to **Mr. Sarthi Soni** for all the advice and wise words he has provided me over the time being. I would like to post my sincere thanks to **Dr Minakshi, Mr. Ganesh, Mr. Dharmendra** for their constant care, support and motivation.

In the end I wish to thank all those who have directly and indirectly contributed to the completion of this dissertation.

Dr. Monika Gupta

CONTENTS

INTRODUCTION

The salivary glands in humans are exocrine glands that produce saliva through a system of ducts. Humans have three paired major salivary glands (parotid, submandibular, and sublingual), as well as hundreds of minor salivary glands [1]. These Structures secreting fluid to facilitate feeding emerge progressively throughout evolution and can be found in very simple organisms and more complex species. In humans, major and minor salivary glands produce and secrete digestive fluids or protein-rich fluids. The three pairs of major salivary glands are responsible for the production and secretion of saliva in the oral cavity, whose moisturizing effect preserves oral hygiene and allows taste, speech and mastication [2]. The parotid gland (PG) is mainly composed of serous acini-secreting α-amylase-rich saliva [3]. The sublingual gland (SL) secretes mucous, a viscous solution rich in mucins [4]. The submandibular gland (SMG) is composed by a mixed population of acini with a mucous and serous function [5]. These three major salivary glands account for more than 90% of salivary secretion. Minor salivary glands are distributed throughout the oral cavity, especially in the labial and lingual mucosa, as well as palate and floor of the mouth. Saliva is an essential fluid for oral cavity maintenance and functionality . Digestive enzymes within saliva initiate the digestion process, and at the same time, saliva acts as a lubricant of solid nutrition, thus helping its passage through the oesophagus . By moisturizing the tongue and other tissues of the oral cavity, saliva has an essential role in speech and taste sensitivity [6]. It also balances the pH of the mouth, thus protecting the soft oral tissues and teeth from an extended exposure to an acidic environment. Saliva contains several signalling molecules, that are essential for the regeneration of oral and oesophageal mucosa. Finally, the antibacterial and antifungal components of the saliva, such as lysozymes, immunoglobulin and lactoferrin, inhibit the progression of bacterial infection and dental caries. Salivary glands play a crucial yet often overlooked role in oral health, and disruptions in their function pose challenges for healthcare professionals.

With diverse aetiologies and presentations, accurate diagnosis of salivary gland disorders is essential. Salivary gland imaging plays a pivotal role in the diagnosis and management of various diseases affecting these glands. From inflammatory conditions to neoplastic lesions, precise imaging modalities help clinicians in characterizing lesions, determining their extent, and guiding appropriate therapeutic strategies. However, selecting the optimal imaging modality tailored to the specific disease of the salivary gland remains a clinical challenge. This protocol aims to streamline the decision-making process by providing guidelines for selecting the most appropriate imaging techniques based on the suspected pathology. By integrating clinical presentation, risk factors, and imaging features, this and endeavours to enhance diagnostic accuracy and facilitate personalized treatment approaches for salivary gland disorders.

OBJECTIVE

This dissertation explores the evolution of salivary gland imaging modalities, examining their utility, advancements, and limitations. Through a comprehensive review of techniques such as ultrasound, Computed Tomography, Magnetic Resonance Imaging, PET, and emerging technologies, we aim to offer a nuanced understanding of their applications in diagnosing various salivary gland pathologies. The rising prevalence of salivary gland diseases necessitates an in-depth investigation into the effectiveness of imaging modalities in characterizing these conditions, from infections and inflammation to neoplasms.

Moreover, understanding the capability of these imaging techniques in distinguishing benign from malignant lesions is crucial for informed decision-making and personalized patient care. This dissertation not only reviews existing literature but also identifies knowledge gaps and potential areas for future research in salivary gland imaging. By critically analysing current modalities' strengths and limitations, we strive to contribute to improved diagnostic protocols and the development of more precise imaging techniques.

Through this comprehensive exploration of the salivary gland imaging landscape, our dissertation aims to provide valuable insights for clinicians, radiologists, and researchers, aiding in the optimization of diagnostic approaches. Ultimately, our goal is to enhance patient outcomes and improve the management of salivary gland pathologies.

MORPHOGENESIS OF SALIVARY GLAND

Salivary glands originate from an epithelial placode during embryonic development (from E11 to E16 between the 4th and the 12th embryonic weeks in humans). The initial placode grows and extends into the underlying mesenchyme, acquiring a bud shape. The growing epithelial bud progressively straits with concentric layers each formed by a specialized cell type. During branching morphogenesis, the initial salivary bud divides into additional, independent buds that grow and cleave again, until the formation of an extensive arborization typical for the mature salivary gland[7].

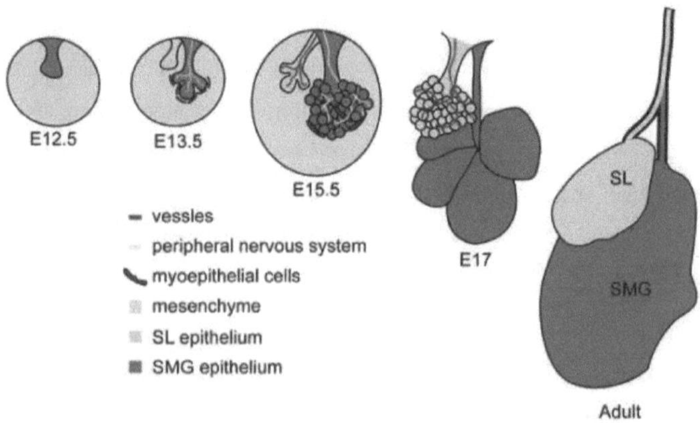

Fig.3.1 Embryonic Development of SMG & SL Gland

A portion of the cells forming the outer epithelial layer of the buds differentiates into myoepithelial cells. They will then acquire smooth muscle characteristics and locate in direct contact with the acinar structure to regulate the release of secretion [8]. Inner epithelial cells differentiate further to acquire a distal (tips) or proximal (stalk) identity, which, in turn, evolves into acini or ducts, respectively [9]. Both epithelial and mesenchymal cells produce the basement membrane and stromal extracellular matrix. The composition of the extracellular matrix varies from region to region during branching, and bundles of collagen I, IV and bronectin are thought to directly control the maturation process.

TYPES OF SALIVARY GLAND

1. Parotid gland

The two parotid glands are major salivary glands wrapped around the mandibular ramus in humans [10]. These are largest of the salivary glands, secreting saliva to facilitate mastication and swallowing, and amylase to begin the digestion of starches [11]. The parotid gland is often described as being divided into superficial and deep lobes by the intraparotid facial nerve and its branches It is the serous type of gland which secretes alpha-amylase (also known as ptyalin). It enters the oral cavity via the parotid duct. The glands are located posterior to the mandibular ramus and anterior to the mastoid process of the temporal bone. They are clinically relevant in dissections of facial nerve branches while exposing the different lobes, since any iatrogenic lesion will result in either loss of action or strength of muscles involved in facial expression [12].They produce 20% of the total salivary content in the oral cavity. Parotid gland saliva is secreted through Stensen's ducts which emerge from the glands, traverse the buccal fat pad superficial to the masseter muscles, and pierce the buccinator muscles to open at papillae in the vicinity of the maxillary first or second molars. Stensen's duct is, on average, between 4 and 6 cm in length and has a diameter between 2.0 and 2.5 mm.

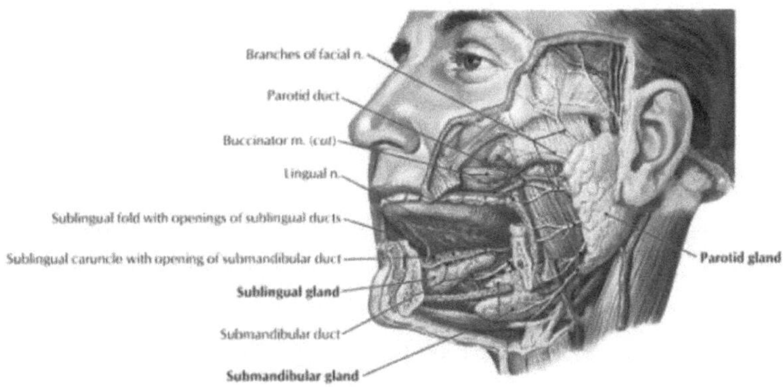

Fig.4.1 Parotid Salivary Gland

2. Submandibular Salivary Gland

The submandibular glands (previously known as submaxillary glands) are a pair of major salivary glands located beneath the lower jaws, superior to the digastric muscles [10]. The secretion produced is a mixture of both serous fluid and mucus, and enters the oral cavity via the submandibular duct or Wharton duct. Each Wharton's duct is approximately 5 cm in length and between 1 and 3 mm in diameter Around 70% of saliva in the oral cavity is produced by the submandibular glands, though they are much smaller than the parotid glands [11].This gland can usually be felt via palpation of the neck, as it is in the superficial cervical region and feels like a rounded ball. It is located about two fingers above the Adam's apple (laryngeal prominence) and about two inches apart under the chin.

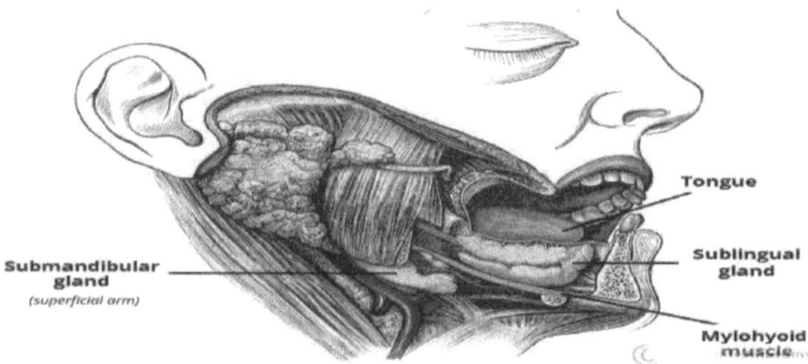

Fig.4.2 Submandibular Salivary Gland

3. Sublingual salivary gland

The sublingual glands are a pair of major salivary glands located inferior to the tongue, anterior to the submandibular glands [10]. The secretion produced is mainly mucous in nature, but it is categorized as a mixed gland. Unlike the other two major glands, the ductal system of the sublingual glands does not have intercalated ducts and usually does not have striated ducts, either, so saliva exits directly from 8-20 excretory ducts known as the Rivinus ducts. About 5% of saliva entering the oral cavity comes from these glands[12].

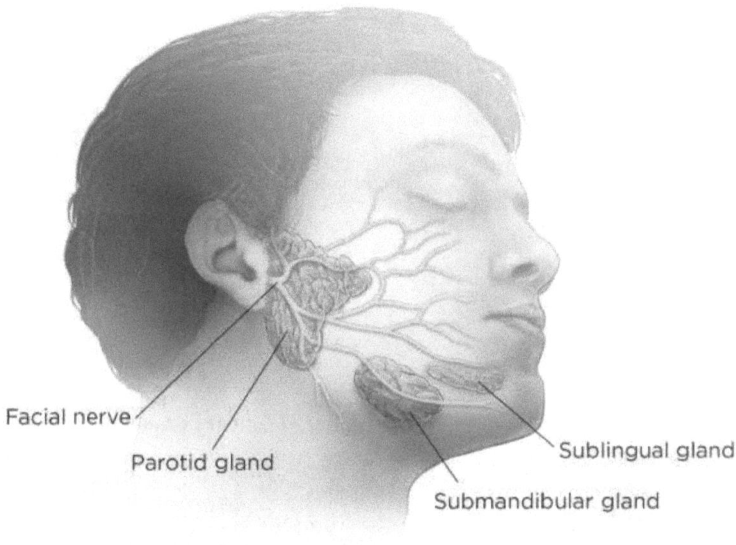

Fig 4.3 Major Salivary Gland

4. **Tubarial salivary gland**

The tubarial glands are suggested as a fourth pair of salivary glands situated posteriorly in the nasopharynx and nasal cavity, predominantly with mucous glands, and its ducts opening into the dorsolateral pharyngeal wall. The glands were unknown until September 2020, when they were discovered by a group of Dutch scientists using with prostate specific membrane antigen PET-CT. This discovery may explain mouth dryness after radiotherapy despite the avoidance of the three major salivary glands. However, these findings from just one study need to be confirmed[13,14].

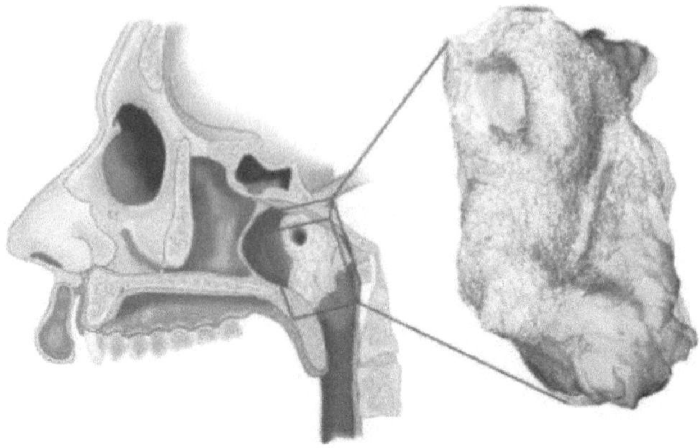

Fig.4.4 Turbarial Salivary Gland

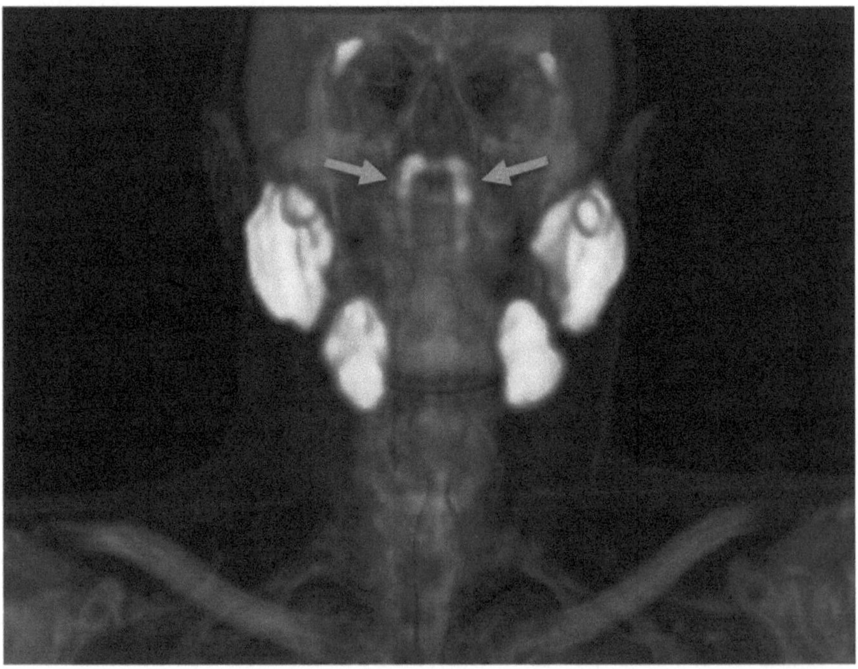

Fig 4.5 Turbarial Salivary gland

There are also three sets of minor salivary glands of the oral tongue: the glands of Weber, found along the lateral borders of the tongue; the glands of von Ebner, surrounding the circumvallate papillae; and the glands of Blandin and Nuhn (also known as the anterior lingual glands), found in the musculature of the anterior ventral tongue. Distinctive mucoceles may arise in the glands of Blandin and Nuhn, highlighting their unique anatomic location.

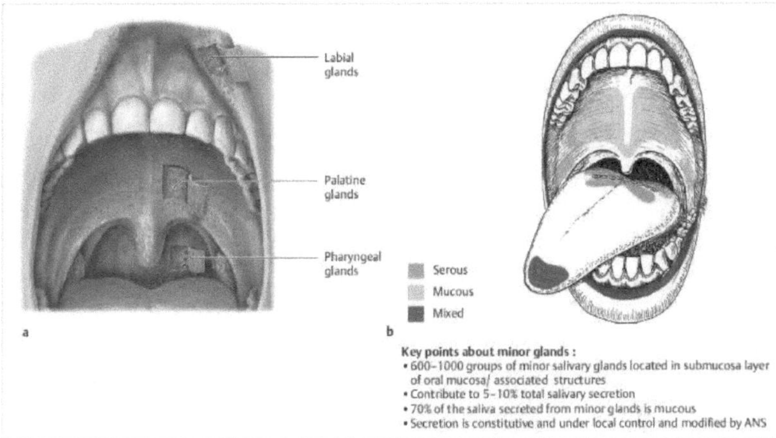

Fig 4.6 shows Minor Salivary Glands

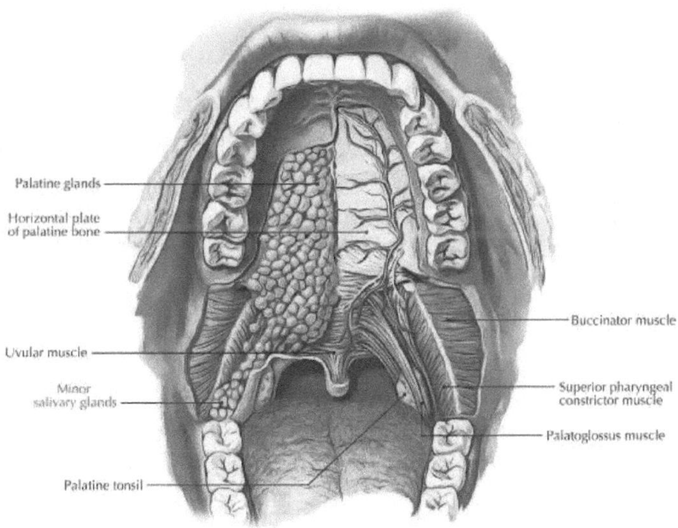

Fig 4.7 shows Minor Salivary Glands

The salivary glands receive innervation from both the autonomic nervous system (ANS) and somatic nervous system (SNS). The innervation plays a crucial role in regulating salivary gland function, including secretion of saliva, blood flow regulation, and sensory feedback. The main nerves involved in the innervation of the salivary glands are as follows:

1. Parasympathetic Nervous System (PNS): Facial Nerve (CN VII): The parasympathetic fibres responsible for salivary gland innervation arise from the superior salivatory nucleus in the pons and travel through the facial nerve (CN VII). These preganglionic fibres synapse in the submandibular ganglion for the submandibular and sublingual glands and in the otic ganglion for the parotid gland.

Glossopharyngeal Nerve (CN IX): Parasympathetic fibres from the inferior salivatory nucleus in the medulla travel through the glossopharyngeal nerve (CN IX) to innervate the parotid gland. These preganglionic fibres synapse in the otic ganglion before reaching the parotid gland.

Functions: Parasympathetic stimulation enhances salivary gland secretion by increasing the production and release of saliva. It also promotes vasodilation, leading to increased blood flow to the salivary glands.

2. Sympathetic Nervous System (SNS):

Sympathetic Trunk (Cervical Sympathetic Chain): Sympathetic Fibers innervating the salivary glands originate from the superior cervical ganglion and travel through the sympathetic trunk. These Fibers primarily regulate blood flow to the glands.

Functions: Sympathetic stimulation leads to vasoconstriction of blood vessels supplying the salivary glands, thereby reducing blood flow. This regulation of blood flow helps modulate saliva production by adjusting glandular perfusion.

3. Somatic Nervous System (SNS):

Trigeminal Nerve (CN V): The mandibular branch of the trigeminal nerve (CN V3) provides sensory innervation to the oral mucosa, including the salivary gland ducts and surrounding tissues. Sensory feedback from these structures helps regulate salivary gland function and plays a role in reflexive responses.

Functions: Somatic sensory innervation mediates sensations such as touch, pressure, and pain in the oral cavity. Sensory feedback from the salivary gland ducts and oral mucosa helps regulate salivary gland secretion in response to stimuli such as taste, chewing, and thermal changes.

Overall, the intricate innervation of the salivary glands by the autonomic and somatic nervous systems allows for precise control of salivary gland function, including saliva production, blood flow regulation, and sensory feedback. Dysfunction or dysregulation of these neural pathways can lead to disorders such as xerostomia (dry mouth), impaired saliva production, or altered sensory perception in the oral cavity.

CHEMISTRY OF SECRETION AND FUNCTION OF SALIVA

Secretion itself is a combination of three events:

(i) nervous cholinergic stimulation initiates uidltration from blood plasma to the acinar lumen.

(ii) exocytosis of cytoplasmic granuli-containing proteins into the acinar lumen.

(iii) mechanical contraction of the secretory end-pieces mediated by specialized myoepithelial cells,

Chemistry of secretion

Primary saliva is initially produced and secreted in acinar cells. Epithelial cells of serous end-pieces are sealed between them via tight junction to preserve apical-basal polarity. This guarantees that electrolytes do not pass freely in between the cells, but require a system of ion-pumps and channels to nely regulate the intracellular and extracellular concentration of each electrolyte. Specially, the Na/K ATPase pumps sodium out of the cell, which then accumulates in the intercellular space. Upon cholinergic stimulus, Ca2+ is released from intracellular storage sites (i.e., ER, mitochondria) and its concentration increases of 5–10-fold in the cytoplasm. This chemical change, in turn, opens the channels for Cl−, which diffuses into the acinar lumen following its concentration gradient. Na+ will then also translocate through the paracellular space to the lumen. Water from the adjacent capillaries will pass into the lumen by osmosis, both through paracellular flow specialized aquaporin channels (mainly AQP5) [15].

Component and Function of saliva -Saliva is a very dilute fluid, composed of more than 99% water. Saliva is not considered an ultrafiltrate of plasma[16]; initially, saliva is isotonic; it is formed in the acini, but it becomes hypotonic when it travels through the duct network. Saliva is 99% water and 1% protein and salts. The normal daily production of saliva varies between 0.5 and 1.5 Liters. The whole unstimulated saliva flow rate is approximately 0.3-0.4 ml / min. This rate decreases to 0.1 ml / min during sleep and increases to about 4, 0-5, 0 ml / min during eating, chewing and other stimulating activities. n adults, normal total stimulated SF ranges 1–3 mL/minute, low ranges 0.7–1.0 mL/minute, while hyposalivation is characterised by a stimulated SF <0.7mL/minute. Quality is checked by Visual Examination-Viscosity

Visually assess the resting viscosity healthy unstimulated saliva is clear in colour and watery in consistency. If it looks stringy, frothy or bubbly, or is very sticky, then it may mean the content of water is low because the rate of production is low.

Salivary component	Function
Amylase and proteases	Digestion
Bicarbonate	Buffering
Calcium	Remineralization
Salivary antibodies and lactoferrin	Antimicrobial
Lysozyme	Hydrolysis of cell membrane
Mucine	Digestion, lubrication and pellicle formation .
Water	Mucosal integrity

Table-5.1 Components of Saliva and its Functions

REVIEW OF LITERATURE

6.1. Salivary Gland Diseases

Salivary glands may be affected by a number of diseases: local and systemic and the prevalence of salivary gland diseases depend on various etiological factors. The glands may be infected by viral, bacterial, rarely fungal or its ductal obstruction which may cause painful swelling or obstruction, affecting their functions. The salivary gland may also be affected by a various benign and malignant tumour.

6.1.2. Classification of salivary gland diseases

TYPES	DISORDERS AND DISEASES
Developmental	Aberrancy, Aplasia, Atresia
Functional	Sialorrhea, Xerostomia
Inflammatory	Chronic sclerosing sialadenitis, Post irradiation sialadenitis
Infectious	Acute bacterial infection, Chronic bacterial infection, Mumps, Viral infection
Obstructive	Mucocele, Mucose retention cyst, Ranula
Traumatic	Sialolithiasis
Autoimmune	Mikulicz disease, Sjogren's syndrome
Degenerative	Idiopathic sialolithiasis
Vascular	Necrotizing sialometaplasis
Benign tumour	Pleomorphic adenoma Warthin tumour Myoepithelioma Basal cell adenoma Lipoma Intercalated duct adenoma
Malignant Tumours	Mucoepidermoid carcinoma Polymorphous adenocarcinoma Histiocytosis X Non-Hodgkin lymphoma with small B cell Acinic cell carcinoma Epithelial-myoepithelial carcinoma

	Salivary duct carcinoma Adenocarcinoma Plasmacytoma
Secondary Tumours	Squamous cell carcinoma Melanoma Baso-squamous carcinoma Trichilemmal carcinoma Infiltrative basal cell carcinoma

Table-6.1 Classification of Salivary Gland Disorders[17]

6.1.3. Various salivary gland disorders

❖ **Developmental Disorders**

1. **Atresia** is the congenital occlusion or absence of salivary ducts which leads to xerostomia or mucous retention cyst.
2. **Aplasia** is the complete absence of one or more salivary gland which leads to xerostomia, and affected patients are more susceptible to dental caries. This condition could be an isolated finding or associated with other disorder like hemi facial microsomia or Treacher Collins syndrome. Recent studies suggest that mutation in fibroblast growth factor 10 (FGF10) affecting the FGF receptor signalling, has been linked with this condition[17]. Enamel hypoplasia, extensive occlusal wear of teeth or congenital absence of teeth are other oral manifestations of salivary agenesis. However, the treatment is supportive.
3. **Aberrancy:** it is an anatomic variant wherein the normal salivary gland develops at an abnormal position. Sometimes they are found adjacent to lingual surface of the mandible within a depression. Ex: Staphne's bone cyst or Staphne's bone cavity: It is thought to be created by an ectopic portion of salivary gland tissue which causes remodelling of the mandibular bone[18]. This lesion is not discovered during routine examination, as it causes no symptoms and do not require intervention. However, surgical intervention is recommended in atypical regions in which the diagnosis is unclear and a tumour is suspected.

❖ **Functional disorders**

1. **Xerostomia**: It is defined as the subjective sensation of oral dryness that may or may not be associated with a reduction in salivary output. The condition may be transient, prolonged or permanent depending upon the duration of the condition.

- Aetiology: Temporary causes are : (1) Psychological causes due to anxiety and depression, (2) Drug Therapy-Drugs that exert anti-anticholinergic and decrease the volume of serous saliva are: anticholinergic, anti-hypertensive, antidepressant anti parkinsonian drugs, anti-emetics. (3) Duct calculi: a blockage of the duct of a major salivary gland (submandibular) can produce dryness on the affected side with pain and swelling in the gland on stimulation. If left untreated it can cause progressive fibrosis of the gland and permanent xerostomia (4) infections, **Sialadenitis** is the inflammation of the salivary gland, acute infections like mumps and post-operative parotitis, chronic conditions like swellings related to nutritional deficiency, and iodine hypersensitivity, wherein in all these conditions causes hypo salivation[19].

  Permanent causes:(5) Salivary gland aplasia, Sjogren's syndrome: causes dry eyes, dry mouth and often associated with rheumatoid arthritis. Other systemic disorders like diabetes mellitus, Parkinson's disease, cystic fibrosis, sarcoidosis, vitamin A, riboflavin, nicotinic acid deficiencies and in anaemia's; (6) Surgery or trauma to the ducts may also impair secretion (7) Radiotherapy: hypo salivation occurs on exposure of major salivary glands to radiation bilaterally in head and neck cancer. At radiation doses > 3000 cGy, the patient is at risk if all major glands are in the field of radiation. Irreversible effects occur at a dose of 6000 cGy for 5 wk. Radiation causes acinar cell atrophy and fibrosis, changes in vascular connective tissue and neurologic function. The degree of salivary gland alteration depends on dose volume factor, patient age, and time of exposure to radiation. Serous acini are affected before mucous acini resulting in thick viscous secretion. Depending on the amount of salivary tissue in the field, xerostomia may resolve within 6 mo. and sometimes may be permanent[20].
- Clinical features: Lips are often cracked, peeling and atrophic; Buccal mucosa may be corrugated and pale:

  (1) Tongue may be smooth and reddened, cracked or fissured, with loss of papillation;

  (2) Increase in erosion and caries, particularly decay on root surfaces and even cusp tip involvement;

  (3) Erythematous form of candidiasis is frequent;

  (4) Lipstick sign: occurrence of shed epithelial cells on the labial surfaces of maxillary anterior teeth as the mucosa adheres to the teeth due to reduced saliva;

(5) Tongue blade sign: when held against buccal mucosa, the tissue adheres to the tongue blade as it is lifted away;

(6) Viscous sticky saliva with difficulty in speaking and swallowing;

(7) Halitosis, altered taste and smell, gingivitis;

(8) Complaint of burning mucosa, lips or tongue;

(9) Ulceration of oral mucosa;

(10) No accumulation of saliva in the floor of the mouth;

(11) Poorly fitting prosthesis; and

(12) Enlargement of salivary glands. Xerostomia associated problems are: Dental Caries, Dry mouth, Dysgeusia, Dysphagia, oral Candidiasis, and Bacterial infections.

- Treatment of xerostomia associated problems: Dental caries; use of fluorinated dentifrice, fluoride gel. Dry Mouth should be hydrated regularly using water or lozenges with citric acid to stimulate salivation, artificial salivary substitutes.

- **Inflammatory**

1. **Sialadenitis** is an inflammation condition affecting the salivary glands. Parotid salivary glands are most commonly affected in adolescents and in children, debilitated adults, or patients with medication on tricyclic antidepressants and tranquilizers.

- Aetiology: The main etiologic factors for sialadenitis can be either infectious or non-infectious factors. Bacterial and viral agents can cause of sialadenitis. Bacterial sialadenitis is caused because of retrograde spread of infection secondary to decreased salivary flow or ductal obstruction. Decreased salivary flow can be secondary to medications, dehydration or debilitating conditions. Ductal obstruction can be due to sialolithiasis, strictures within the ductal system and common in submandibular salivary glands or due to pressure effect from adjacent tumours. Staphylococcus aureus is the most common etiologic agent for acute bacterial parotitis in addition Staph. Pyogenes, Strep. Viridians and other microorganisms can also cause sialadenitis. Viruses causing sialadenitis include paromyxo viruses (mumps-most common), Coxsackie virus, cytomegalo virus, etc. The patient may present with fever and dehydration[21].

- Clinical features: clinically there is sudden pain at the angle of the jaw which is unilateral with glandular enlargement and tender to palpation with purulent discharge over Stenson's duct.
- Treatment includes administration of salivary stimulants, antibiotics and surgical drainage.

2. Acute postoperative parotitis

- Aetiology is a form of sialadenitis which occurs after a major surgical procedure where in the patient depends only on intravenous fluids. In addition, these patients are on atropine which is a pre anaesthetic medication for drying the secretions and this may contribute to dryness of mouth and subsequent inflammation of parotid salivary glands. Non-infectious causes of salivary gland inflammation are sarcoidosis and Sjogren's syndrome.
- Clinical features: Parotid gland is the most common salivary gland involved in acute bacterial sialadenitis. The patient presents with painful, usually bilateral swelling of the parotid salivary glands with low grade fever. In addition, the patient may also complain of difficulty in opening the mouth. On clinical examination the skin over the parotid region may be inflamed and intra orally purulent discharge may be observed from parotid duct.
- Treatment-The condition usually resolves in about 48 h. However, symptomatic treatment is recommended.

o **Mumps** is an acute paramyxo virus induced infection of parotid salivary glands.

- Aetiology- It is a contagious infection spreading through airborne droplets or direct contact of saliva. The peak incidence of mumps is reported during winter and spring season[18].
- Clinical features: The infectivity of the mumps virus ranges from 3 to 4 d after the onset of the disease[19]. During the prodromal phase of the disease, the patient may complain of low-grade fever, muscle pain, head ache and malaise, followed by unilateral or bilateral enlargement of parotid salivary glands associated with pain which is severe during mastication. The inflammation of the salivary gland starts reducing by the end of 1st week and the patient returns to normal by 10 days[19].
- Treatment is symptomatic and Mumps vaccination (MMR) may decrease the incidence of this infection and considered as preventive measure.

3. **Chronic recurrent parotitis**

- The proposed etiopathogenesis for this disorder include, congenital[20,21] and acquired factors like ductal obstruction secondary to inflammation infection and autoimmune diseases[22].

4. **Chronic sclerosing sialadenitis:** Also known as Kuttner's tumour was identified by Kuttner in 1896.

- Aetiology-The condition is a chronic inflammatory reaction secondary to ductal obstruction and subsequent salivary stasis. However, salivary flow obstruction is proposed to be the main factor in the pathogenesis of this disorder [23].
- Clinical feature: Clinically the condition presents as a painful, hard swelling of submandibular salivary gland. The pain and swelling may be present for a variable duration of time. The differential diagnosis includes chronic sialadenitis, sialolithiasis, and benign lymphoepithelial lesions.
- Treatment-The condition is managed by surgical excision of the involved gland and chances of recurrence of the lesion or changing into malignancy is found to be rare [23].

5. **Hepatitis c virus associated sialadenitis:**

- Aetiology-hepatitis C virus (HCV) is found to affect the salivary glands and cause the glandular inflammation.
- Clinical feature: The affected patients may present with mild swelling of the parotid gland with minimum or no symptoms of dry eyes and dry mouth [24].
- The diagnosis of HCV is by the detection of HCV DNA and anti HCV antibodies.
- Treatment- Hepatitis associated sialadenitis is treated symptomatically.

6. **Human immunodeficiency virus infection:** In Human immunodeficiency virus (HIV) infected patient's salivary gland lesions commonly occur which may be neo plastic or non-neoplastic in nature. AIDS related tumours such as lymphoma and Kaposi's sarcoma and a Sjogren's syndrome like condition occurs in these patients and are described as ―HIV salivary gland disease‖ (HIV-SGD) is considered to be due to reactivation of a latent virus. Various studies have expressed the strong association between salivary gland dysfunction seen in HIV affected patients and Human Cytomegalovirus (CMV) saliva[24].

- Clinical feature: The condition is characterised by xerostomia with unilateral or bilateral salivary gland enlargement with reduced tear production.
- Diagnosis is by biopsy of the major gland which shows the presence of hyperplastic lymph nodes with lymphocytes and cystic cavities obtained from patients affected from HIVSGD.
- Treatment-Administration of oral sialagogues/ frequent sipping of water are recommended for xerostomia. Anti-retroviral therapy may be administered for the management of HIV. Rarely radiotherapy and parotidectomy may be beneficial in advanced condition.

7. **Iodine 131 induced sialadenitis:**

- Aetiology-high dose of oral Iodine 131 in treatment of thyroid carcinomas can adversely affect the salivary glands leading to sialadenitis. The incidence of acute salivary gland inflammation ranges from 24%-67% and that of chronic salivary gland inflammation range from 11%-43%[25.26].
- Clinical feature: The patients present with pain and swelling of the salivary glands with or without dry mouth condition.
- Treatment- Administration of oral sialagogues/oral hydration, serotonin receptor blocker and dexamethasone are recommended.

8. **Sialadenosis:** Sialadenosis also known as sialosis is an enlargement of salivary glands which is non-inflammatory and non-neoplastic more commonly affecting the parotid salivary glands.

- Aetiology: This condition can be associated with: Endocrine disorders: (1) Diabetes mellitus and insipidus; (2) Acromegaly; (3) Hypothyroidism; and (4) Pregnancy. Nutritional status: (1) Anorexia nervosa; (2) Bulimia; (3) Chronic alcoholism; and (4) General malnutrition. Medication induced sialadenosis[27]: (1) Psychotropic medications; (2) Antihypertensive drugs; and (3) Sympathomimetic drugs.
- Clinical features- Patient presents with a slowly progressing bilateral (rarely unilateral) swelling of parotid salivary glands which may be asymptomatic[28]. Rarely patients may complain of reduced salivary flow.
- Treatment-Management of underlying systemic condition may help in reversing the sialdenosis.

❖ **Traumatic**

1. **Mucocele**

   ➢ Aetiology-They is caused due to rupture of a salivary gland duct mostly due to trauma resulting in spillage of mucin into the surrounding tissues.

   ➢ Clinical features: Clinically a mucocele appear as bluish thin-walled lesion which is fluctuant, and the most common site of occurrence is on the lower lip. Ranula: is a special type of mucocele which grows in the floor of the mouth, usually unilateral and is called due to its similar appearance to enlarged abdomen region of a frog.

   ➢ Treatment-in case of superficial recurrent or deep mucoceles, surgical intervention is indicated while large ranulas are treated by marsupialization. A study by Wilcox et al[29] recommends intra lesional corticosteroids administration before surgery.

2. **Nicotinic stomatitis**:

   ➢ Aetiology-The long-standing habits of tobacco and or alcohol/hot liquid consumption. Clinical feature: Exhibits whitened areas of the hard palate due to hyperkeratosis caused by the thermal irritation. This irritation also causes inflammation and dilatation of the duct openings of the minor salivary glands of the palate manifesting as red patches or spots on a white background[29].

   ➢ Treatment- discontinuation of the habits reverses the condition back to normal

❖ **Autoimmune:**

1. **Sarcoidosis**

➢ Aetiology-is an autoimmune chronic granulomatous inflammatory condition which causes destruction of the tissue by T lymphocytic, mononuclear phagocytic infiltration and granuloma formation[29]. The parotid salivary glands are affected in 10%-30% of cases.

➢ Clinical feature: The patient presents with a hard, bilateral enlargement of the parotid gland usually asymptomatic in nature. Sarcoidosis of parotid glands along with uveitis and facial nerve paralysis is termed as Heerfordt's syndrome or uveo parotid fever. The patient may complain of dry mouth and minor salivary gland biopsy confirms the diagnosis.

➢ Treatment-palliative treatment primarily relieving of the symptoms of salivary component of sarcoidosis is advised. Corticosteroid or with Chloroquine has been recommended. Immunosuppressive and immune modulatory medications are administered in patients who do not respond the corticosteroids.

2. **Sjogren's syndrome**

- Aetiology-is an autoimmune disorder associated with HLA-DR3 AND HLA-B8. The disease was described by Henric Sjogren in 1933.
- Clinical feature: The primary Sjogren syndrome/sicca complex exhibit dry eyes and mouth. The secondary Sjogren syndrome develops SLE, polyarteritis nodosa, polymyositis, rheumatoid arthritis and in scleroderma. This condition is most commonly seen in women over 40 years with male: female in the ratio of 1: 10. Sjogren's syndrome case definition[28] requires at least 2 out of the following 3 criteria as mentioned-
  - Positive serum anti-SSA and/or anti-SSB or (positive rheumatoid factor and ANA $\geq$ 1:320)
  - Ocular staining score ≥ 3
  - Presence of focal lymphocytic sialadenitis with focus score $\geq$ 1 focus/4 mm2 in labial salivary gland biopsies
- Laboratory findings: Anti salivary duct antibodies, anti-nuclear antibodies, rheumatoid factor increased ESR, Lip biopsy-lymphocytes around salivary glands. The other tests are Schirmer test, Rose Bengal dye test, Sialography and sialo chemistry.
- Treatment to limit the harmful effects of the disease especially the ocular and oral conditions, symptomatic relief of administration of artificial tears, saliva substitutes, fluoride applications and oral hygiene measures are suggested[28].

3. **Mikulicz's disease**

- Aetiology-Mikulicz's disease of unknown aetiology was first reported by Johann von Mikulicz-Radecki in 1888. However, it has been demonstrated that autoimmune, viral, and genetic factors may contribute to the pathogenesis of the disease.
- Clinical feature: Patients suffering from Mikulicz's disease present with asymptomatic, bilateral swelling of the parotid, and submandibular salivary glands along with lacrimal glands. This disease closely resembles Sjogren's syndrome. However, the lacrimal and salivary secretion depletion is very minimal in Mikulicz's disease. Histologically the disease resembles Sjogren's syndrome, but lacks the characteristic anti-SS-A and anti-SS-B antibodies of Sjogren's syndrome.

Studies have found increased levels of IgG4 antibodies in the serum of patients with Mikulicz's disease[30].

- Treatment- Mikulicz' s disease is very much responsive for steroid therapy particularly to methylprednisolone.

- **Neurological**

1. **Frey's syndrome** also known as Auriculo temporal syndrome which is characterized by sweating in the pre auricular and temporal areas after gustatory stimulation.

- Aetiology-the condition most commonly caused due to faulty regeneration of sympathetic and parasympathetic nerve fibres which were injured during parotid tumour surgery or ramus resection.
- Clinical feature: Post-surgery the parasympathetic fibres start innervating the sweat glands and vasculature of the skin around the parotid area. The symptoms usually appear within few minutes of the start of mastication or during stimulation of saliva and may remain up to 30 min after discontinuing mastication. The diagnosis of the syndrome can be confirmed by starch iodine test[31].
- Treatment- Reassurance to the patient is advocated in most of the cases. Intra cutaneous injection of botulin toxin is found to be effective in severe condition and Tympanotomy[21] may be the treatment of choice with severe symptoms.

- **Degenerative**

1. **Sialolithiasis**-is a condition of unknown aetiology. However, there could be several coexisting causes leading to the salivary stone formation. Some of these cofactors may be related to disturbed pH of saliva, abnormalities in the sphincter mechanism related to salivary duct opening and abnormal calcium metabolism[29].
   - Clinical Feature: This condition most often will not produce any signs and symptoms. Rarely, it may cause complete ductal obstruction, pain and swelling of the salivary glands.
   - Treatment- Large salivary stone are managed by extracorporeal or intracorporal lithotripsy procedure.

- **Non inflammatory non neoplastic**

1. **Sialadenosis** is a non-infectious, non-inflammatory gland enlargement usually affecting the parotid bilaterally. This condition is most often seen in women causing salivary hypo salivation which can occur due to systemic disorders[32].

- **Vascular**

1. **Necrotizing sialo metaplasia**

- Aetiology-The probable cause could be due to vascular infarction of the salivary gland lobules and is often mistaken for oral cancer[33]. Vascular compression is caused by a necrotic Myo cutaneous reconstruction of the flap used in palatal surgeries and embolization from carotid endarterectomises, Berger' s disease, Raynaud's phenomenon. Predisposing factors are dental injections, ill-fitting denture, traumatic injury, previous surgery and upper respiratory tract infections.
- Clinical feature: appears as a non-neoplastic lesion that usually arises from a minor salivary gland in the lips, posterior part of the palate, and retro molar regions.
- Treatment: The condition is self-limiting and the healing of the lesion normally takes about 6-8 wk.

- **Neoplastic**

1. **Benign:** Pleomorphic Adenoma, Papillary Cystadenoma Lymphomatosum (Warthin's tumour), Basal Cell Adenomas, Oncocytoma, Canalicular Adenoma, Myoepithelioma, Sebaceous Adenoma, Ductal Papilloma.

   Benign salivary gland tumours are neoplasms originating from the glandular tissue of the salivary glands. These tumours can arise from any of the major salivary glands (parotid, submandibular, and sublingual glands) or the numerous minor salivary glands located throughout the oral cavity, pharynx, and upper respiratory tract. Some common benign salivary gland tumours include:

   1. Pleomorphic Adenoma (Benign Mixed Tumour):

   Pleomorphic adenoma is the most common benign salivary gland tumour, accounting for approximately 60-70% of all salivary gland neoplasms. It typically arises from the parotid gland but can also occur in the submandibular gland or minor salivary glands.

   Pleomorphic adenoma is characterized by a mixture of epithelial and mesenchymal components, including ductal epithelial cells, myoepithelial cells, and stromal elements. Histologically, it exhibits a biphasic pattern with epithelial and mesenchymal components.

Clinical Features-Pleomorphic adenoma usually presents as a slow-growing, painless, well-circumscribed mass in the parotid or other salivary glands. It may be mobile and firm to palpation.

Treatment-Surgical excision is the primary treatment for pleomorphic adenoma. Complete removal with clear margins is essential to prevent recurrence.

2. Warthin Tumour (Papillary Cystadenoma Lymphomatosum):

Warthin tumour is the second most common benign salivary gland tumour, frequently occurring in the parotid gland. It is more common in males and often presents in the 5th to 7th decades of life.

Warthin tumour is characterized by cystic spaces lined by bilayered epithelium and surrounded by lymphoid stroma. It often contains oncocytic epithelial cells and lymphoid tissue.

Clinical Features-Warthin tumour typically presents as a painless, slow-growing mass in the parotid gland. It may be associated with smoking and has a predilection for multicentricity.

Treatment-Surgical excision is the treatment of choice for Warthin tumour. The recurrence rate following complete excision is low.

3. Monomorphic Adenoma (Basal Cell Adenoma, Canalicular Adenoma):

Monomorphic adenoma is a relatively uncommon benign salivary gland tumour, accounting for a small percentage of salivary gland neoplasms. It can arise from the parotid, submandibular, or minor salivary glands.

Monomorphic adenoma is characterized by a uniform population of epithelial cells with minimal stromal components. It may exhibit tubular, trabecular, or cribriform growth patterns.

Clinical Features-Monomorphic adenoma typically presents as a painless, slow-growing mass in the affected salivary gland. It is usually well-circumscribed and may have a rubbery consistency.

Treatment-Surgical excision with clear margins is the mainstay of treatment for monomorphic adenoma. Recurrence rates are low with complete resection.

4. Oncocytoma:

Oncocytomas are rare benign salivary gland tumours composed predominantly of oncocytic cells. They can arise from the parotid gland, submandibular gland, or minor salivary glands.

Oncocytomas are characterized by large, eosinophilic, granular cells with abundant mitochondria. These cells form solid nests or acinar structures within a fibrous stroma.

Clinical Features-Oncocytomas usually present as painless, slow-growing masses in the affected salivary gland. They are often well-circumscribed and may exhibit a tan or brown coloration on cut section.

Treatment-Surgical excision is the primary treatment for oncocytomas. Complete removal with clear margins is essential to prevent recurrence.

Other benign tumours include adenolymphomas, myoepitheliomas, basal cell adenomas, and cystadenomas, among others. Each tumour type has distinct histological features, clinical presentations, and management approaches. Early detection, accurate diagnosis, and appropriate treatment are essential for optimal outcomes in patients with benign salivary gland tumours.

2. Malignant: Adenoid Cystic Carcinoma, Hyalinising Clear Cell Carcinoma, Mucoepidermoid Carcinoma, Acinic Cell Carcinoma, Adeno carcinoma, Pleomorphic Adenoma, Lymphoma [29].

Malignant salivary gland tumours, also known as salivary gland carcinomas, arise from the epithelial cells of the salivary glands and can occur in both major (parotid, submandibular, sublingual) and minor salivary glands (located throughout the oral cavity and upper aerodigestive tract). These tumours exhibit a wide range of histological subtypes, each with distinct clinical and pathological characteristics. Here are some of the most common malignant salivary gland tumours:

1. Mucoepidermoid carcinoma is the most common malignant salivary gland tumour, comprising a heterogeneous mixture of mucinous, epidermoid (squamous), and intermediate cell types. It typically arises in the parotid gland but can occur in other salivary glands as well. Mucoepidermoid carcinoma may exhibit low, intermediate, or high-grade histology, with varying clinical behaviour and prognosis.

2. Adenoid cystic carcinoma is a slow-growing malignancy characterized by cribriform and tubular growth patterns, along with the presence of basaloid cells and hyaline stroma. It commonly arises in the submandibular gland and minor salivary glands, often presenting with perineural invasion and a propensity for local recurrence and distant metastasis.

3. Acinic cell carcinoma is characterized by serous acinar cell differentiation and typically presents as a well-circumscribed, encapsulated mass. It commonly arises in the parotid gland but can occur in other major and minor salivary glands. Acinic cell carcinoma typically exhibits low to intermediate-grade histology and has a favourable prognosis compared to other malignant salivary gland tumours,

4. Salivary Duct Carcinoma (SDC), formerly known as salivary duct adenocarcinoma, is an aggressive malignancy characterized by ductal differentiation and histological resemblance to ductal carcinoma of the breast. It commonly arises in the parotid gland and exhibits high-grade histology, often associated with rapid growth, lymphovascular invasion, and distant metastasis.

5. Adenocarcinoma, Not Otherwise Specified (NOS): Adenocarcinoma NOS is a heterogeneous category encompassing various subtypes of adenocarcinomas that do not fit into specific diagnostic categories. These tumours may exhibit glandular or papillary growth patterns and are associated with variable clinical behaviour and prognosis depending on histological features and tumour grade.

6. Carcinoma ex pleomorphic adenoma refers to a malignant transformation of a pre-existing pleomorphic adenoma, the most common benign salivary gland tumour. This transformation can give rise to various malignant histological subtypes, including mucoepidermoid carcinoma, adenoid cystic carcinoma, acinic cell carcinoma, and carcinoma ex pleomorphic adenoma (CEPA) itself.

Other rare subtypes include epithelial-myoepithelial carcinoma, salivary myoepithelial carcinoma, basal cell adenocarcinoma, and clear cell carcinoma, among others. Treatment strategies for malignant salivary gland tumours typically involve surgical resection, often followed by adjuvant radiation therapy or chemotherapy, depending on the histological subtype, tumour stage, and patient factors. Early detection, accurate histological diagnosis, and multidisciplinary management are crucial for optimizing outcomes in patients with these tumours.

6.2 SALIVARY GLAND IMAGING

Diagnostic imaging plays an important role in the management of patients presenting with signs and symptoms related to the major salivary glands. Imaging may be useful in assessing the nature of the abnormality, the extent of involvement, the effects on the adjacent anatomic structures, and possibly, the causes.

The imaging modalities are helpful to have a better insight and orientation about salivary gland disorders. They are useful adjuncts to clinical examination for diagnosing salivary glandular pathology. The following are the imaging modalities used for salivary gland imaging[34]:

1. Plain Film Radiography
2. Ultrasonography
3. Sialography
4. Computed tomography (CT)
5. Magnetic Resonance Imaging (MRI)
6. Nuclear Medicine
7. Sialendoscopy

6.2.1 Plain film radiography

Plain film radiography gives two-dimensional information about three dimensional objects, but, object localization techniques like right angled technique helps in viewing the pathology in two different angulations giving an idea about the third dimension. However, with plain film radiography, the overlapping of anatomic structures around the region of interest cannot be avoided. The plain radiographic techniques for parotid gland are Puffed cheek Anteroposterior (AP) view, buccal soft tissue intraoral radiograph, Lateral oblique (Ramus-Condyle) view. The radiographic techniques for submandibular/sublingual gland are Lateral oblique view with the tongue depressed, mandibular occlusal view and over the shoulder occlusal projection view[35].

Projection images, whether intraoral occlusal images or extraoral panoramic images, are helpful in identifying calcified sialoliths. Cross-sectional mandibular occlusal images are best used to identify submandibular duct sialoliths[36], whereas panoramic images may be used to demonstrate both parotid and submandibular sialoliths. Parotid sialoliths appear superimposed over the mandibular rami superior to the occlusal plane, whereas submandibular sialoliths appear superior to the hyoid bone near the ante gonial notch of the mandible[37]. Therefore, these images should be considered first when the patient presents with signs and symptoms suggestive of a sialolith such as swelling and pain just prior to or during mealtime[37]. Some of the advantages of projection images are that they are readily available, are inexpensive, and subject the patient to a relatively low dose of radiation. In addition, they allow examination of osseous structures adjacent to the salivary glands[38]. However, projection images do fail at identifying noncalcified sialoliths, which are estimated to account for 40% of all parotid sialoliths and 20% of all submandibular sialoliths[39].

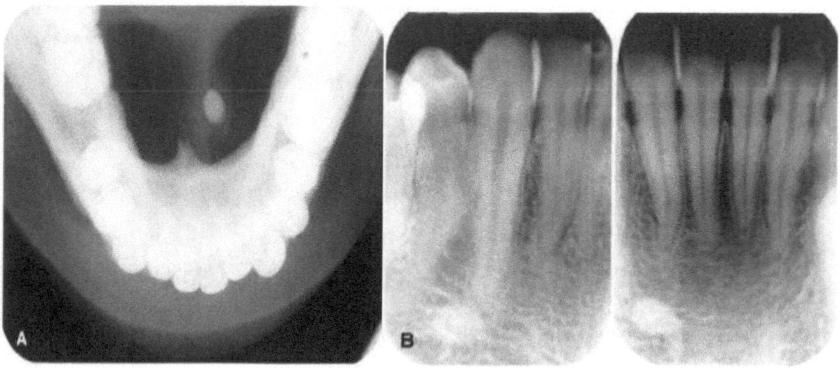

Fig. 6.2.1 shows (A) Standard mandibular Occlusal, (B) periapical imaging demonstrating an oval- shaped radiopaque sialolith in a Wharton duct

Plain radiography, particularly panoramic radiography, is commonly employed as an initial diagnostic tool for detecting sialoliths. It demonstrates a sensitivity ranging from 54% to 84% and specificity of approximately 85% to 100%[40]. Plain radiography can aid in the diagnosis of acute sialadenitis by demonstrating ductal dilation and parenchymal changes. However, its sensitivity and specificity in this condition are relatively low compared to other imaging modalities such as ultrasound and MRI[41]. Plain radiography may reveal calcifications or soft tissue masses suggestive of neoplasms in the salivary glands. However, its sensitivity and specificity are limited, and it is primarily used as an adjunctive tool to other imaging modalities such as CT and MRI[42].

Advantages of Plain Radiography:

- Widely available and cost-effective.
- Low radiation exposure compared to CT scans.
- Useful for initial screening and follow-up assessments.

Disadvantages of Plain Radiography:

- Limited sensitivity and specificity, especially in detecting smaller lesions and soft tissue abnormalities[43].
- Inability to provide detailed anatomical information compared to CT or MRI.
- Overlapping structures may obscure findings.

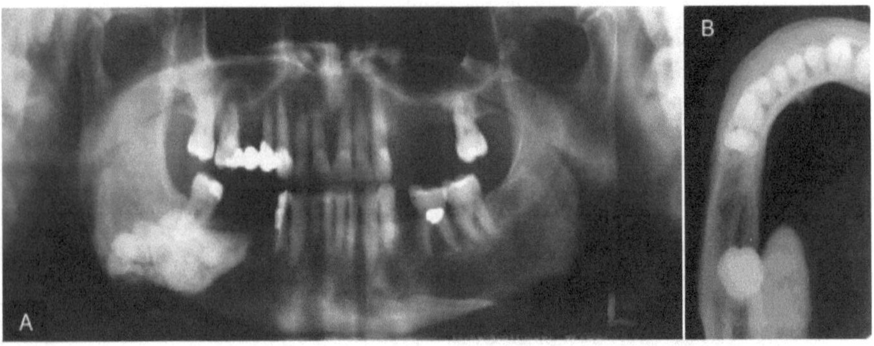

Fig 6.2.2 shows Panoramic radiograph (A) and asymmetric mandibular occlusal radiograph (B) of the same patient demonstrating a large calcified sialolith in the right submandibular gland duct. Both images can be used to detect calcified sialoliths and to assess the surrounding osseous structures.

6.2.2 High resolution Ultrasonography

It is an ideal first line investigatory imaging modality for major salivary glands. It is useful to investigate the pathologies intrinsic and extrinsic to the salivary glands. Since it doesn't use ionizing radiation, it is an appropriate chairside procedure to detect the presence of salivary glandular pathology. Non-invasive and widely available. Utilizes high-frequency sound waves to produce images of the salivary glandsThis technique may be used for the initial assessment of the parotid and submandibular glands, both glands appear homogeneously hyperechoic on HRUS, and retromandibular vein can be noted within the parotid gland [Fig 6.2.3]. especially when an abnormality is located superficially. It may also be used to guide biopsies and further imaging choices. HRUS is helpful at differentiating cysts from neoplasms, and benign from malignant lesions [Fig 6.2.4]. HRUS has become more specific at detecting Sjögren syndrome, but it is still lacking in its ability to detect sialoliths. The major disadvantage of HRUS lies in its inability to detect deep salivary gland lesions.

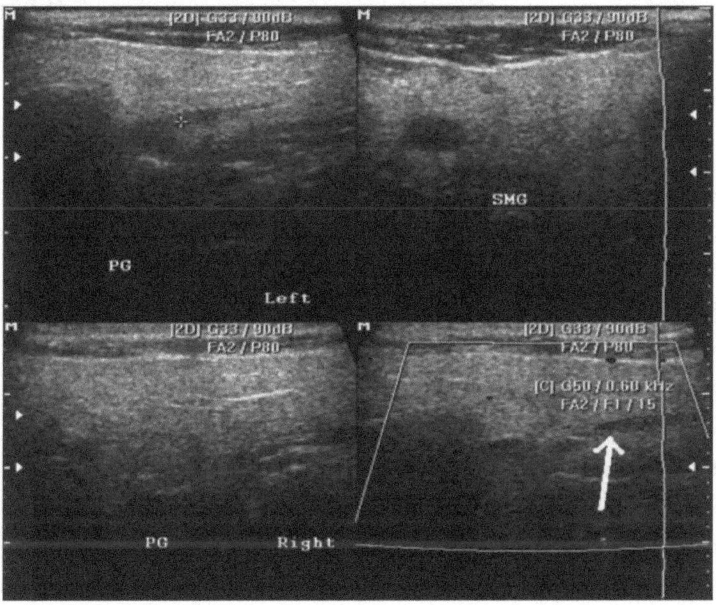

Fig 6.2.3 High-resolution ultrasonography images showing normal parotid and submandibular glands (top row) and retromandibular vein in the parotid gland (arrow)

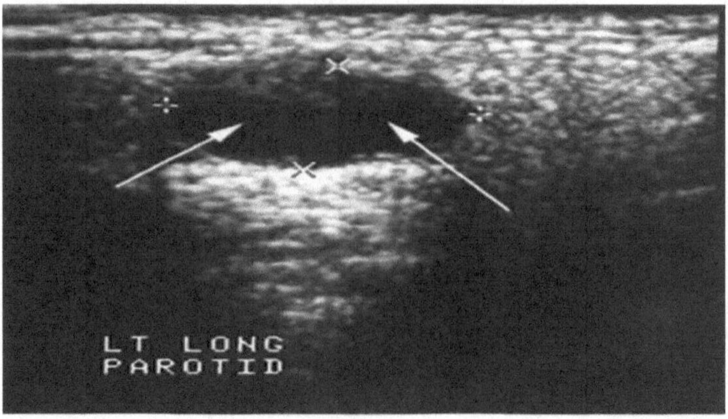

Fig 6.2.4 High-resolution ultrasonography image of the parotid gland demonstrating an echo-free mass with well-defined margins, which is typical of a cystic mass (arrows)

It can be combined with FNAC to diagnose salivary glandular diseases. Some studies have documented the utility and safety of Ultrasound Guided Fine Needle Aspiration of Salivary gland masses and found the sensitivity of this modality to be 93.7%. Other studies have given a sensitivity value of 80% and specificity values of 95% for FNAC in parotid glandular lesions. A non-diagnostic rate of 10% is documented by some studies. Fine needle aspiration biopsy (FNAB) is an alternative modality to FNAC in diagnosing salivary gland diseases. It found the sensitivity values of FNAB to be 96% (95% confidence interval (CI) = 87–99%) and the specificity values were found to be 100% (95% CI = 84~100). Colour Doppler technique helps in the diagnosis of salivary gland diseases by assessing the vascularity of the lesion. The malignant salivary gland tumours tend to be more vascular than the benign salivary gland tumours. Pleomorphic adenoma, the commonest salivary gland neoplasm, is characterised by peripheral vascularity with central hypo vascular area. RI>0.7 and PI>1.2 along with PSV > 44.3 cm/s, ill-defined margins, nodal involvement with central vascularity are highly indicative of a malignant salivary gland lesion[44,45].

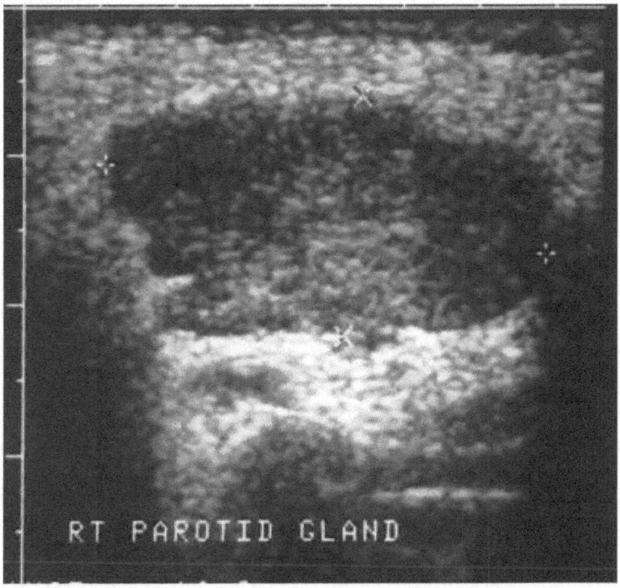

Fig 6.2.5 shows s a solid mass in the superficial lobe of right parotid gland

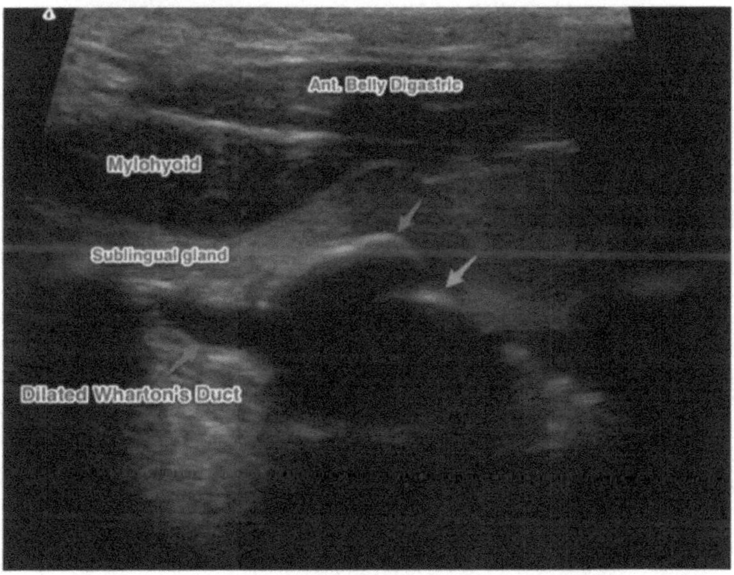

Fig 6.2.6 shows Ultrasound of the right submandibular/floor of the mouth region

USG demonstrates high sensitivity and specificity in detecting salivary gland disorders, with reported values ranging from 85% to 95% for sensitivity and 90% to 98% for specificity [44,46].

1. Sialolithiasis: USG is the initial imaging modality of choice for detecting salivary gland calculi due to its high sensitivity and specificity. It allows for precise localization and characterization of calculi within the salivary ducts, aiding in treatment planning[47,48,60].

2. Sialadenitis: USG is valuable in diagnosing acute and chronic sialadenitis, demonstrating gland enlargement, parenchymal heterogeneity, and ductal dilation. Doppler USG can assess vascularity, aiding in differentiating infectious from non-infectious causes[49,50,61].

3. Sialadenosis: USG helps evaluate diffuse enlargement of salivary glands seen in sialadenosis, revealing symmetric gland hypertrophy without discrete masses[51]. It assists in ruling out neoplastic processes and guiding further management.

4. Salivary Gland Tumours: USG serves as a primary imaging tool for detecting and characterizing salivary gland neoplasms, differentiating cystic from solid lesions[52]. It provides valuable information on lesion size, location, and relationship with adjacent structures, aiding in preoperative planning [53,62].

5. Sjögren's Syndrome: USG plays a role in diagnosing Sjögren's syndrome by detecting characteristic glandular changes such as hypoechoic areas, glandular heterogeneity, and loss of normal architecture[54]. It helps assess disease severity and guide biopsy site selection for histological confirmation[55].

6. HIV-related Salivary Gland Diseases: USG assists in evaluating HIV-related salivary gland diseases, including lymphoepithelial cysts and lymphadenopathy, demonstrating chacteristic sonographic features [56]. It aids in differentiating benign from malignant lesions and monitoring disease progression.

7. Postoperative Complications: USG is valuable in detecting postoperative complications such as hematoma, seroma, and abscess formation following salivary gland surgery, guiding appropriate intervention[57]. It enables early detection and management, minimizing morbidity and improving patient outcomes.

8. Radiotherapy-related Changes: USG can detect radiation-induced changes in salivary glands, including glandular atrophy, fibrosis, and ductal dilation, assisting in monitoring treatment response[58]. Longitudinal USG evaluations help assess treatment-related complications and guide supportive care strategies.

9. Autoimmune Disorders: USG aids in diagnosing autoimmune disorders affecting salivary glands, such as IgG4-related disease, by demonstrating diffuse gland enlargement with hypo echogenicity and peri glandular halo[59]. It assists in differentiating autoimmune conditions from neoplastic processes and monitoring disease activity.

Advantages of USG:

- Non-invasive and readily available.
- Cost-effective compared to other imaging modalities like MRI.
- Provides real-time imaging, aiding in dynamic assessments.
- Can differentiate between cystic and solid lesions, aiding in diagnosis[63].

Disadvantages of USG:

- Operator dependence may affect accuracy.
- Limited ability to evaluate deep-seated lesions or lesions obscured by bone structures.
- Lower resolution compared to MRI for detailed tissue characterization[64].

6.2.3 Multidetector Computed Tomography (MDCT)

MDCT, displayed in both hard- and soft-tissue windows, is useful in evaluating not only the salivary glands but also the structures surrounding them [Fig. 6.2.5]. This is especially true when the images are acquired after intravenous administration of a contrast agent that renders glandular tissues hyperdense relative to the surrounding fat and muscle[42]. MDCT imaging is used in cases when inflammation of the salivary glands is suspected because it demonstrates characteristic features such as peripheral enhancement, thickening of the subcutaneous tissue, and lymph node involvement, some or all of which can be seen in inflammation or neoplasia. Sialoliths are well depicted on MDCT images but only if they are relatively large and significantly calcified. Smaller, less-calcified sialoliths and ductal strictures are not well[65,66].

Unfortunately, CT alone cannot differentiate benign from malignant masses because benign masses have capsules that give them a smooth well-defined contour when imaged and low-grade malignancies have pseudo capsules that can also give them a smooth well-defined outline. Fortunately, when CT findings are combined with clinical findings, the distinction between benign and malignant masses can be made in 90% of cases. With regard to obstructive conditions, CT demonstrates large calcified sialoliths with great sensitivity but fails to demonstrate small and non-calcified ones and it fails to show the ductal changes that result from chronic obstruction.

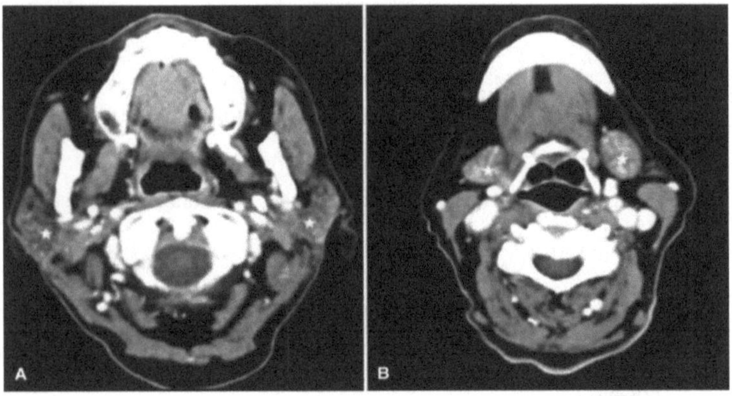

Fig 6.2.7 shows Axial soft-tissue algorithm multidetector computed tomography images (A) at the level of the parotid glands (stars) and (B) at the level of the submandibular glands (stars). Because the salivary glands have fatty stroma than muscles, they appear less dense than adjacent muscles

CT imaging demonstrates high sensitivity and specificity in detecting salivary gland abnormalities, with reported values ranging from 80% to 95%. CT is particularly valuable in evaluating the size, location, and extent of lesions within the salivary glands[66].

1. Sialolithiasis: CT imaging is considered the gold standard for detecting salivary gland stones due to its high spatial resolution and ability to visualize calcifications. It exhibits sensitivity and specificity exceeding 90%[67].

2. Sialadenitis: CT aids in the diagnosis of acute and chronic sialadenitis by demonstrating glandular enlargement, peri glandular inflammation, and abscess formation. Its sensitivity and specificity range from 85% to 95%[67].

3. Salivary Gland Tumours: CT imaging assists in characterizing salivary gland tumours based on their size, margins, and tissue attenuation. While it provides valuable preoperative staging information, its sensitivity and specificity vary depending on tumour histology[68].

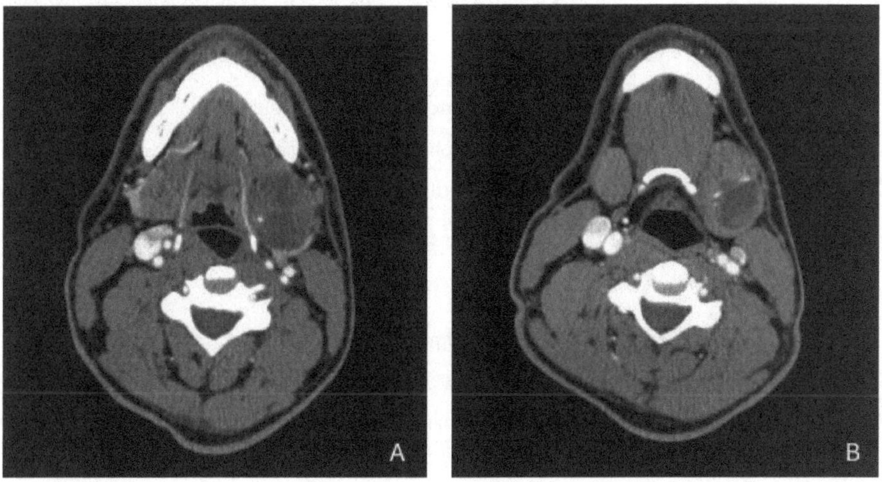

Fig 6.2.8 shows Computed tomography (CT) images of the left submandibular gland. Soft tissue algorithm axial CT images at the level of the mandible (A) and at the level of the submandibular region (B) demonstrating a well-defined, expansile lesion within the gland with an internal homogeneous low attenuation.

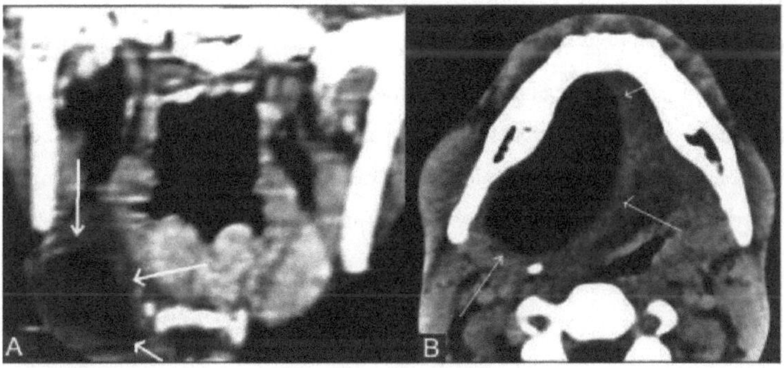

Fig 6.2. shows Contrast-enhanced coronal CT image (A) shows submandibular mucocele on right side (thick white arrow) while axial CT image (B) shows right sublingual gland mucocele (thin white arrows)

Comparison of CT, CBCT, and MDCT: CBCT offers high spatial resolution and reduced radiation dose compared to conventional CT, making it advantageous in dental applications such as evaluating parotid gland involvement in dental pathologies[69-71]. MDCT provides faster acquisition times and improved temporal resolution, enabling dynamic contrast-enhanced imaging for assessing salivary gland perfusion and vascularity.

Advantages of CT Imaging:

- Provides detailed anatomical information and spatial relationships.
- Offers multiplanar reconstruction capabilities, enhancing diagnostic accuracy.
- Rapid acquisition times and widespread availability contribute to its utility in clinical practice.

Disadvantages of CT Imaging:

- Limited soft tissue contrast compared to magnetic resonance imaging (MRI).
- Ionizing radiation exposure, especially in paediatric and young adult populations.
- Suboptimal visualization of small lesions, particularly in the setting of adjacent bony structures.

6.2.4 Magnetic Resonance Imaging

Although indications for MRI occasionally overlap with those of MDCT, MRI is the imaging method of choice for assessment of space- occupying lesions (cyst and neoplasms) of the salivary glands because of its superior soft-tissue contrast [Fig.6.2.5]. In addition, the use of intravenous gadolinium as a contrast agent makes MRI the imaging modality of choice for evaluation of intracranial and perineural spread of disease[72,73]. Detection of sialoliths, particularly when calcified, is problematic in MRI because these calcific entities result in signal voids. Other disadvantages of MRI include long acquisition times, relatively poor spatial resolution, cost, and accessibility[74].

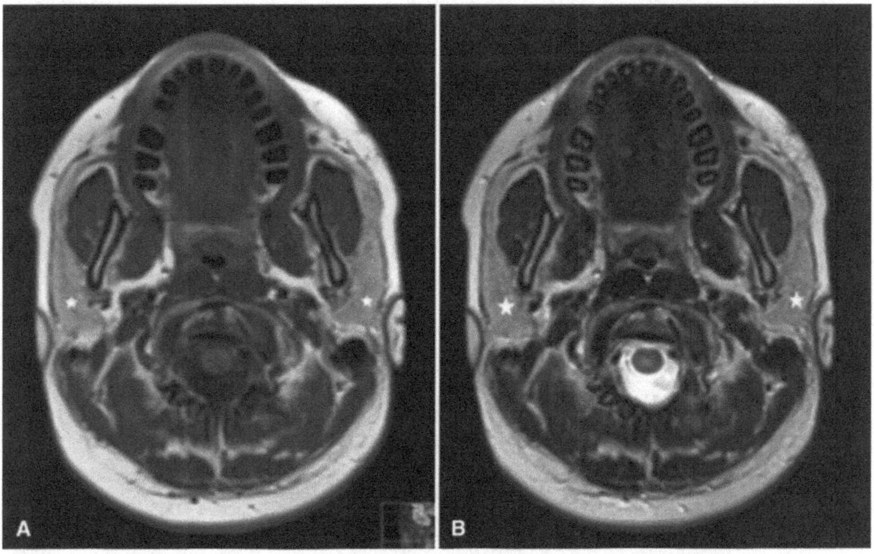

Fig 6.2.9 shows Magnetic resonance imaging of normal parotid glands. (A) T1- weighted image and (B) T2-weighted image displaying the hyperintense signal of the parotid glands (stars) relative to the adjacent muscle.

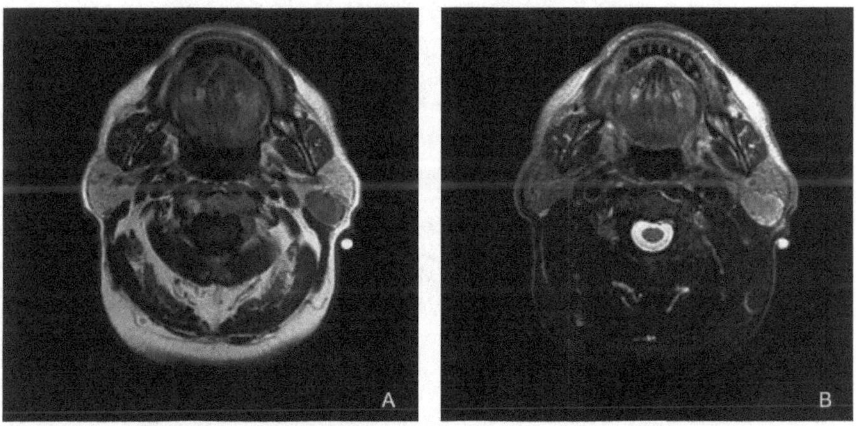

Fig 6.2.10 shows Magnetic resonance images (MRI) of the left parotid gland. Axial T1 weighted MR image (A) and T2 weighted MR image (B) of the left parotid gland demonstrating a mass in the tail of the gland. The mass has a low T1 signal and a higher T2 signal which is suggestive of a benign neoplasm

1. Sialadenitis: MRI aids in the differentiation of acute and chronic sialadenitis, with a sensitivity of 92% and specificity of 100%. It accurately depicts glandular enlargement, inflammation, and abscess formation[75].

2. Sialolithiasis: MRI demonstrates excellent sensitivity (95-100%) and specificity (93-100%) in detecting salivary gland calculi. It provides detailed anatomical localization and characterization of stones[76].

3. Sjögren's Syndrome: MRI aids in assessing salivary gland involvement, demonstrating sensitivity ranging from 72% to 100% and specificity from 82% to 100%. It reveals glandular atrophy, heterogeneous enhancement, and periductal fibrosis[77].

4. Salivary Gland Tumours: MRI is the imaging modality of choice for characterizing salivary gland tumours, with sensitivity and specificity exceeding 90%. It accurately delineates tumour size, location, and involvement of adjacent structures[78].

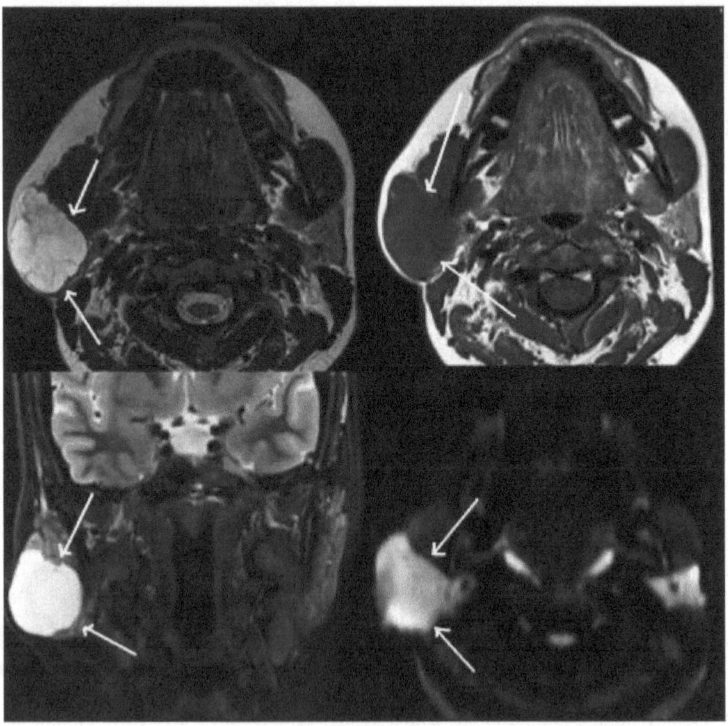

Figure 6.2.11: shows non-contrast T2 & T1W axial images (upper row) and T2W coronal & DW axial images (lower row) show pleomorphic adenoma of right parotid gland (white arrows)

5. Autoimmune Sialadenitis: MRI demonstrates sensitivity ranging from 81% to 95% and specificity from 85% to 100% in diagnosing autoimmune sialadenitis. It reveals diffuse glandular enlargement, heterogeneous enhancement, and periductal inflammation[79].

6. Mucoceles: MRI demonstrates sensitivity ranging from 85% to 100% and specificity from 88% to 100% in diagnosing mucoceles. It depicts cystic lesions with low signal intensity on T1-weighted images and high signal intensity on T2-weighted images[80].

7. Salivary Duct Obstruction: MRI demonstrates sensitivity ranging from 85% to 100% and specificity from 88% to 100% in diagnosing salivary duct obstruction. It reveals ductal dilatation, proximal glandular enlargement, and secondary inflammatory changes[81].

8. HIV-Related Salivary Gland Disease: MRI demonstrates sensitivity ranging from 76% to 92% and specificity from 86% to 100% in detecting HIV-related salivary gland disease. It reveals glandular enlargement, heterogeneous enhancement, and periductal lymphocytic infiltration[82].

9. Radiation-Induced Sialadenitis: MRI demonstrates sensitivity ranging from 81% to 95% and specificity from 85% to 100% in diagnosing radiation-induced sialadenitis. It reveals glandular atrophy, heterogeneous enhancement, and periductal fibrosis[83].

Advantages of MRI-

- High soft tissue resolution allows for precise characterization of inflammatory changes.
- Non-invasive imaging modality with multiplanar capability for comprehensive evaluation
- Allows for early detection and monitoring of disease progression
- Allows for early detection and monitoring of disease progression
- Allows for accurate differentiation of cystic lesions
- Provides detailed anatomical information for guiding therapeutic interventions.
- Allows for early detection and monitoring of radiation-induced complications.
- Non-invasive and radiation-free
- High sensitivity and specificity in detecting salivary gland pathologies

Disadvantages of MRI-

- Costly compared to some imaging modalities
- Limited availability in certain regions
- Claustrophobia may limit patient compliance
- Artifact susceptibility in the presence of metal implants
- Limited specificity in distinguishing between infectious and non-infectious aetiologies
- Limited sensitivity in detecting small calculi, especially in the submandibular gland duct
- Limited ability to differentiate between benign and malignant lesions based solely on imaging features

These cross-sectional studies help in true and near complete imaging of the salivary glands [Figures 6.2.11 and 6.2.12]. MRI, because of its multiplanar capability and higher soft tissue resolution, has an upper hand over CT in demonstrating the extent of lesion and their perineural/meningeal spread. However, CT (especially cone-beam CT) demonstrates the osseous lesions/extension and calcification/calculus better than MRI. Noncontract CT may be enough in cases of sialolithiasis. However, ductal system is not optimally evaluated by any of these techniques.

These studies are often performed after intravenous injection of the contrast media for better delineation of the anatomy and the extent of lesion. Diffusion-weighted (DW) images and gadolinium-enhanced dynamic MR (Gd-MRI) imaging have proven to be very useful in differentiating benign from malignant tumours.[84,85] DW images can be used to calculate apparent diffusion coefficient (ADC) values, which are different for different salivary gland tumours. Gd-MR with dynamic imaging using 120 s as cut-off for time to peak enhancement and 30 % wash-out ratio can differentiate benign and malignant tumours as the latter take less time for peak enhancement and show rapid wash-out. Plateau type of time–intensity curve in dynamic Gd-MR coupled with low ADC values is also highly suggestive of malignancy. Proton MR Spectroscopy has also been described for differentiation of benign from malignant tumours by some authors. Choline/creatinine ratios are significantly lower in malignant than in benign salivary gland tumours[86] .

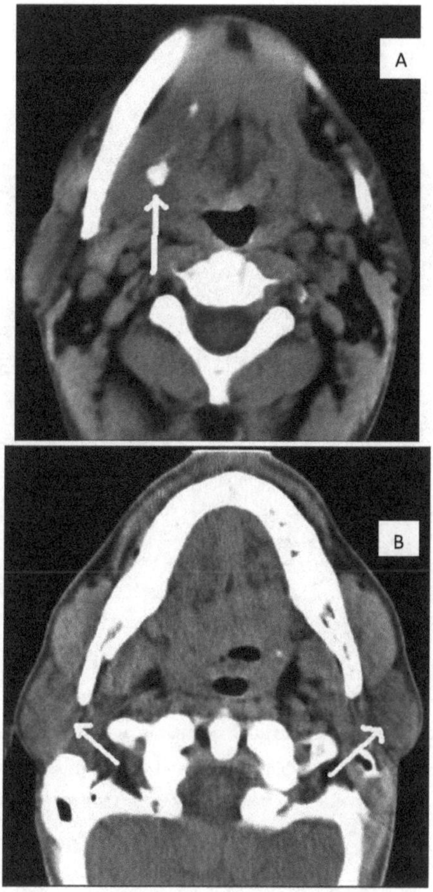

Fig 6.2.12 shows (A)Non-contrast axial CT image showing submandibular sialolithiasis on right side (white arrow) and normal gland on left side (B) Non-contrast axial CT image show normal appearing parotid (white arrows) gland in a young subject

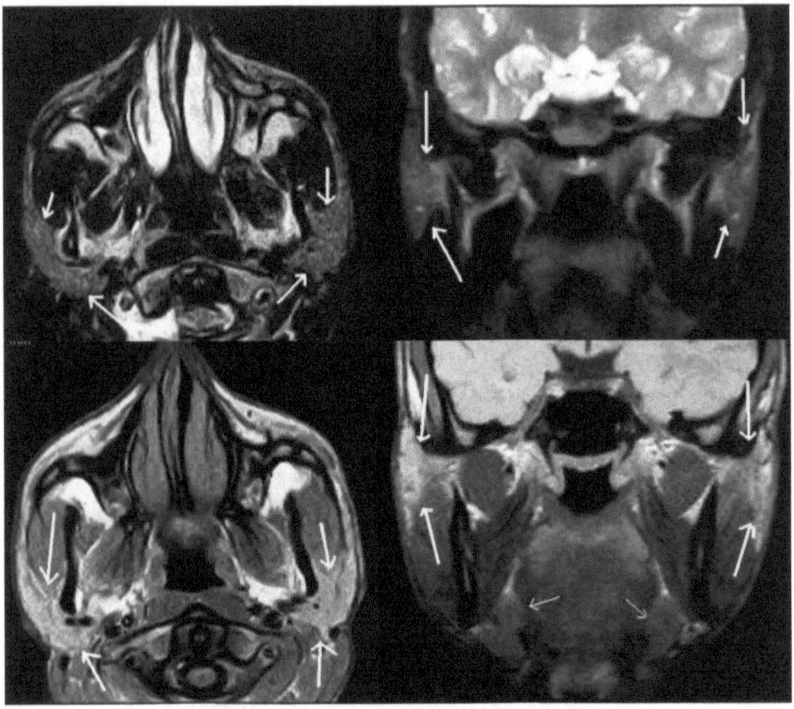

Fig 6.2.13 shows non-contrast T2W axial & coronal images (top row) and T1W axial and coronal images showing parotid (thick white arrows) and submandibular glands (thin white arrow)

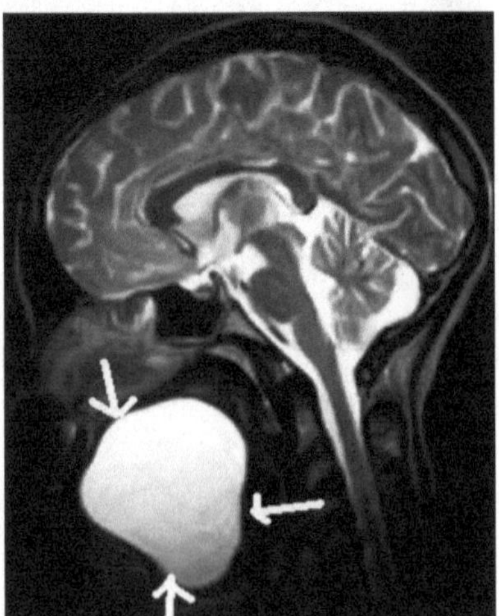

Figure6.2.14: T2W sagittal MR image shows a sublingual epidermoid cyst (white arrows)

6.2.5 Sialography

First performed in 1902, sialography is an imaging technique exclusively used for the parotid and submandibular salivary glands. The technique involves infusion of the gland ductal system with an iodinated contrast agent, and then imaging the gland with projection imaging, fluoroscopy, MDCT, or cone beam computed tomography (CBCT). Sialography is the only imaging technique that can assess both the morphology of the parotid and submandibular glands in addition their function. The rate of clearance of the contrast agent from the gland, especially when prolonged, is used as an indirect indicator of reduced secretory function. The primary indication for sialography is chronic inflammatory conditions, especially when obstruction is suspected[88]. There are two contraindications for sialography. The first of these is acute infection because injection of the contrast agent may disperse the infection into otherwise unaffected regions within the gland and cause further pain for the patient[88]. The second contraindication is an immediately anticipated thyroid function test because the iodine in the contrast agent may concentrate in the thyroid gland and interfere with the results of the test.

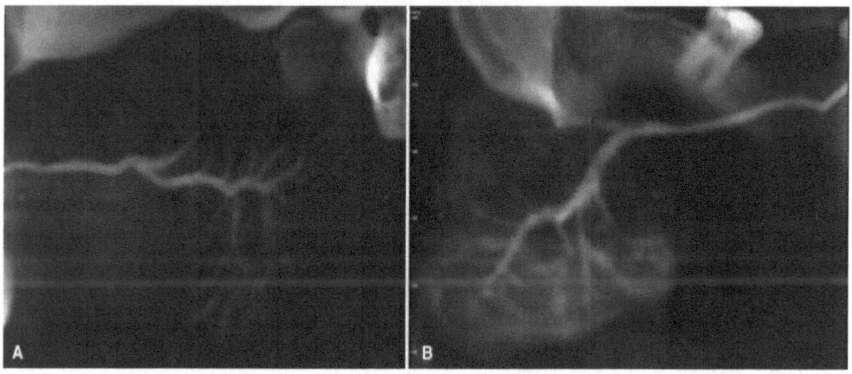

Fig 6.2.15 shows Sialography coupled with cone beam computed tomography. (A) Corrected sagittal image of a normal left parotid gland illustrating the branching pattern of the ductal structures. (B) Corrected sagittal image of a normal right submandibular gland also illustrating the branching ducts. The outline of the gland body is displayed here due to filling of the acini with contrast material

Conventional Sialography and Digital Subtraction Sialography

Conventional sialography requires the technical ability to dilate and cannulate a salivary duct orifice as well as skill in radiographic assessment with fluoroscopy. Although it is more readily performed than —minimally invasivel diagnostic sialendoscopy. Sialography may be considered not only diagnostic but also therapeutic in some cases. The process of distal duct dilation with catheter insertion as well as hydro-dilation of the entire system with —flushing out the glandl employs a radiocontrast water-soluble iodinated compound that has bactericidal activity [89]. Tucci et al. in 2019 reported successful treatment of juvenile recurrent parotitis in 89% of 110 patients (all younger than 16 years of age) employing sialography without local anaesthesia or sedation [90]. These investigators suggested that sialography —broke the cycle of decreased secretion, stasis and infectionl by improving duct patency with cannulation, instilling iodine-based (antiseptic) radiocontrast, and flushing out debris and epithelial plugs in the duct and gland. Sialography has additionally been useful in guiding procedures performed within the ductal system under fluoroscopic control. These procedures have been reported to include salivary stone lithotripsy, stone extraction, and balloon ductoplasty [91].

Use of subtraction imaging as is commonly applied to digital subtraction angiography (DSA) is designed to highlight perfused vessels and digitally remove the appearance of overlapping structures to improve image interpretation. When applied to sialography, this subtraction imaging requires stabilization of the head to ensure that pre-contrast images (mask images) are taken in the identical position as those following intraductal contrast infusion (live images). Computer processing removes the mask image (subtraction) from the live image(s) in an effort to eliminate the view of soft tissue and bony structures to focus on the detail of ductal anatomy in two dimensions [92,93,96]. Unfortunately, there is some degree of —spatial inconsistency between the two images caused by inevitable and complex motion of patientl resulting in blurring from motion artifact [94]. This —interscan motionl is of greater concern in the course of dynamically manipulating the catheterized salivary duct than with the intravascular infusion done during angiography performed in an immobilized patient. Conventional sialography in the distant past was performed in an —analoguel manner that required —analogue to digital conversionl when subtracting mask images to result in —digital subtraction sialographyl [95]. Conventional sialography is now done with enhanced digital recording in a manner that, with the addition of improved (more dense) radiocontrast agents and technical considerations including optimal head positioning, has negated the value in performing subtraction. In similar fashion, although CT sialography had found advocates in the past, the loss of detail in ductal definition when compared to contemporary —conventionall sialography—coupled with the increased radiation exposure of CT imaging—has made this imaging option less useful. The capacity to assess ductal changes in an unlimited number of orientations employing the —fourth dimensionl (time) that is available with conventional sialography is lost when only several images (usually pre-, intra-, and post-insufflation) are available as with CT sialography [97]. Fluoroscopic salivary duct imaging has additionally been used to direct procedures such as interventional basket retrieval for proximal, mobile stones [98]. Reports of complication from sialography in the past have included concern about extravasation of radiocontrast (—duct rupturel) that has been negated as a concern by use of absorbable water-soluble radiocontrast. Despite employing pliable plastic Angio catheters to cannulate the salivary ducts, Truong et al. still reported a 4.7% radiocontrast ductal extrusion rate among 255 sialograms reviewed [99]. These investigators identified in each case the extravasation was associated with ductal stricture and had no associated complications as the water-soluble contrast material was readily absorbed.

MR Sialography MR sialography was developed to evaluate the salivary ducts by employing a special technique of heavily T2- weighted rapid acquisition with relaxation enhancement to exploit the imaging potential of the high T2 signal intensity of stationary fluids [100]. The capacity to image the main salivary ducts without instilling contrast (saliva within the ducts acts as the contrast media) makes MR sialography useful for those patients whose ducts cannot be cannulated due to scarring or other reasons. MR sialography has gained support for evaluation of obstructive sialadenitis due to its capacity to image the main salivary ducts [101-103]. Additional disadvantages to use of MR sialography include the standard general patient contraindications for MRI and image artifact due to dental fillings, implants, or amalgam.

CT Sialography and Cone Beam CT Sialography In a manner similar to conventional sialography, both CT and CBCT sialography are performed after ductal cannulation and contrast injection. However, this modality remains mainly a diagnostic tool to help guide therapeutic procedure, and not used concurrently with intervention [104,105]. CT sialography is capable of demonstrating both soft tissue and glandular parenchyma in addition to ductal anatomy. Moreover, three-dimensional reconstruction can be performed with CBCT to offer additional perspective in orientation [106].

6.2.6 Nuclear Medicine

Nuclear medicine examinations are functional examinations of the salivary glands. This modality takes advantage of the selective uptake of specific radiopharmaceuticals such as technetium 99m (99mTc)-pertechnetate (TPT) by the salivary glands when injected intravenously. This is followed by administration of a sialagogue to evaluate the secretory capacity of the salivary glands. Pathosis may be determined on the basis of variations in the rate of TPT uptake or clearance. For example, Warthin tumour distinctively demonstrates reduced TPT clearance. Nuclear medicine is a highly sensitive technique that allows examination of all the major salivary glands at once; however, it lacks specificity and resolution which makes assessment of the salivary gland morphology difficult.

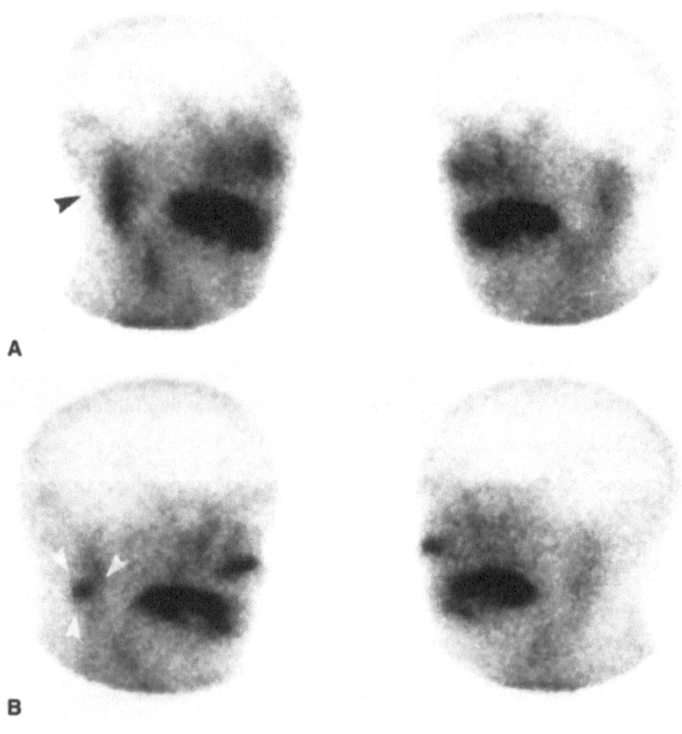

Fig 6.2.16 shows Nuclear Medicine. (A) Technetium 99m (99mTc)-pertechnetate (TPT) scan of the salivary glands (right and left anterior oblique views) demonstrates increased uptake in the right parotid gland (black arrowhead). (B) Nuclear medicine image obtained after administration of a sialagogue (lemon juice) demonstrates retention of TPT in the right parotid gland (white arrowheads). This is a typical presentation of a Warthin neoplasm.

Radionuclide Imaging

Scintigraphy is also a functional examination of the major salivary glands with the added advantage of being able to examine all the major salivary glands at once. scintigraphy is a radiologic examination that does not examine the morphologic anatomy but rather the physiologic function of a tissue or organ. Scintigraphy is also known as radionuclide imaging because it uses a radioactive molecule that emits gamma rays. When injected intravenously, the radiopharmaceutical distributes in the body and is selectively concentrated by certain tissues. Then when it starts to decay, a solid-state scintillation camera is used to detect gamma emissions. Glandular tissues including the thyroid and salivary glands uptake, concentrate, and excrete the radiopharmaceutical technetium-99m (99mTc) pertechnetate (TPT). Technetium-99m (99mTc) is a metastable isotope of technetium with a short half-life of 6 hours, and pertechnetate is the water-soluble ion that carries and distributes it in the body. In the salivary glands the concentration of TPT reaches a maximum at about 30 to 45 minutes.6 A sialagogue (lemon juice) is then administered to assess the excretory function of the glands. Lesions are identified through either an increased, decreased or absent uptake and excretion of TPT. Certain salivary gland tumours, namely Warthin's tumours and oncocytomas characteristically concentrate TPT. Scintigraphy of the 30 salivary glands like all other nuclear medicine imaging studies has high sensitivity but low specificity which in addition to its low resolution limits its clinical applicability.

1. Sialadenitis: Imaging Technique: Technetium-99m pertechnetate (99mTc) scintigraphy. Sensitivity Specificity: Sensitivity ranging from 77% to 92%, specificity up to 90%[107].

- Advantages: Non-invasive, functional evaluation, assessment of salivary gland function
- Disadvantages: Limited spatial resolution, radiation exposure

2. Sialolithiasis: Imaging Technique: Salivary gland scintigraphy with 99mTc. Sensitivity/Specificity: Sensitivity varies from 81% to 95%, specificity up to 90%[108].

- Advantages: Detection of small stones, functional assessment, differentiation from other causes of gland enlargement
- Disadvantages: Limited anatomical localization, false positives in inflammatory conditions

3. Sjögren's Syndrome: Imaging Technique:* PET with fluorine-18-fluorodeoxyglucose (18F-FDG). Sensitivity/Specificity: Sensitivity ranging from 82% to 93%, specificity up to 95%[109].

- Advantages: Detection of metabolic activity, assessment of disease extent, early detection of lymphoma transformation
- Disadvantages: Limited availability, false positives in inflammatory conditions

4. Salivary Gland Tumours: Imaging Technique: 99mTc sestamibi scintigraphy. Sensitivity/Specificity: Sensitivity varies from 76% to 94%, specificity up to 90%[110]

- Advantages: Evaluation of tumour uptake, differentiation of benign and malignant lesions
- Disadvantages: Limited spatial resolution, false negatives in small tumours

5. Radiation-Induced Salivary Gland Dysfunction: Imaging Technique: Salivary gland scintigraphy with 99mTc. Sensitivity/Specificity: Sensitivity ranging from 73% to 88%, specificity up to 95%[111]

- Advantages: Functional assessment of glandular damage, monitoring treatment response.
- Disadvantages: Radiation exposure, limited anatomical detail

6. Mucocele: Imaging Technique: Technetium-99m pertechnetate (99mTc) scintigraphy. Sensitivity/Specificity: Sensitivity ranging from 80% to 90%, specificity up to 95%[112].

- Advantages: Functional evaluation, differentiation from other cystic lesions
- Disadvantages: Limited spatial resolution, false positives in inflammatory conditions

7. Ranula: Imaging Technique: Technetium-99m pertechnetate (99mTc) scintigraphy. Sensitivity. Specificity: Sensitivity ranging from 75% to 88%, specificity up to 92%[113]

- Advantages: Functional assessment, differentiation from other cystic lesions
- Disadvantages: Limited spatial resolution, false positives in inflammatory conditions

8. Salivary Gland Infections: Imaging Technique: Technetium-99m pertechnetate (99mTc) scintigraphy. Sensitivity/Specificity: Sensitivity ranging from 79% to 92%, specificity up to 88%[114]

- Advantages: Functional assessment, differentiation from non-infectious causes
- Disadvantages: Limited anatomical detail, false positives in inflammatory conditions

9. Salivary Gland Trauma: Imaging Technique: Salivary gland scintigraphy with 99mTc. Sensitivity/Specificity: Sensitivity ranging from 74% to 85%, specificity up to 90%[115]

- Advantages: Functional evaluation, assessment of glandular damage
- Disadvantages: Limited spatial resolution, false positives in inflammatory conditions

10. Recurrent Pleomorphic Adenoma: Imaging Technique:Technetium-99m pertechnetate (99mTc) scintigraphy. Sensitivity/Specificity: Sensitivity ranging from 78% to 92%, specificity up to 90%[116].

- Advantages: Functional assessment, detection of recurrent disease.
- Disadvantages: Limited spatial resolution, false positives in inflammatory conditions

6.2.7 Sialendoscopy

Since its first use in the 1990s, this examination that involves direct visualization of the parotid and submandibular major ducts (has transformed the diagnosis and management of obstructive conditions of these glands. The minimally invasive technique can be equipped with sialolith retrieval and stricture dilation tools that have enabled management of these common conditions with reported success rates greater than 95%. Acute inflammation is the only known contraindication for this relatively new technique because of the possible pain that may be elicited[117].

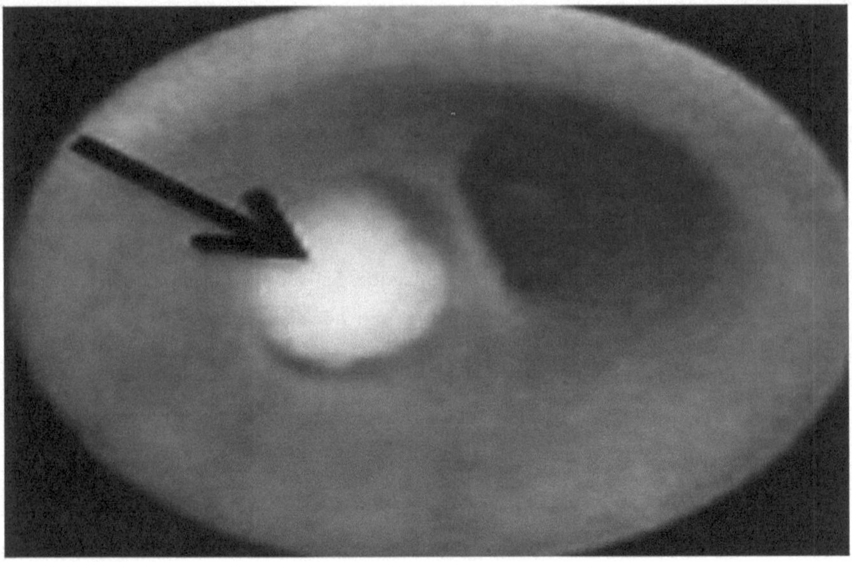

Fig 6.2.17 shows Sialendoscopy allows direct visualization of the salivary gland ducts. This particular image demonstrates a sialolith (arrow) in one of the branching ducts

Emerging imaging-based diagnostics: Positron emission tomography (PET) scan: A PET scan focuses for areas of high cellular activity suggesting a sign of cancer growth. It also helps to diagnosed cancer, and to assess its spread to lymph nodes or any other parts of the body. Positron emission tomography (PET) imaging using 2-deoxy-2-[18F] fluoro-d -glucose (FDG) can be used to differentiate benign from malignant tumours of the salivary glands as the former appear as cold spots with the exception of Warthin's tumour and oncocytoma.[118].

This test requires an injection of a very small quantity of radioactive substance usually a type of sugar known as FDG, which will be excreted by the body later in a day. As cancer cells growth is faster in the body, they absorb more of the radioactive sugar. After about an hour, the patient is moved onto a table and made to lie for about 30 min. Meanwhile a special camera captures a picture of areas of radioactivity in provide helpful information about whole body. It is also possible to take a PET and CT scan at the same time (PET/CT scan). This enables the doctor compare areas of higher radioactivity on the PET scan with the more detailed picture of that particular area on the CT scan.

DISCUSSION

Imaging plays a crucial role in the diagnosis and management of salivary gland disorders, including sialolithiasis, neoplasms, infections, and inflammatory conditions. Various imaging modalities offer distinct advantages and limitations in assessing these disorders, and the choice of modality depends on factors such as the suspected pathology, clinical presentation, and availability of resources.

1. Congenital Lesions of salivary gland

These include cysts (type I branchial cyst, salivary cysts, dermoid, and epidermoid cysts), lipoma, haemangioma, lymphangioma, sialo lipoma, and sarcoma .Majority occur in the parotid glands and some of them such as lipoma, haemangioma, dermoid cyst, and lymphangioma. Various modalities can be used for imaging these lesions, including ultrasound, computed tomography (CT), magnetic resonance imaging (MRI), and salivary gland scintigraphy. In terms of sensitivity and specificity, MRI is generally considered the best imaging modality for evaluating congenital lesions of the salivary gland due to its superior soft tissue contrast and lack of ionizing radiation. However, more studies are required to find out which imaging modality is best suitable for congenital lesions of salivary glands.

2. Functional Disorders of Salivary gland

Salivary Gland Scintigraphy (SGS) SGS is a nuclear medicine imaging technique used to evaluate salivary gland function. SGS can assess both qualitative and quantitative aspects of salivary gland function, including glandular uptake, distribution, and clearance of the radiotracer. It has relatively high sensitivity and specificity in detection the functional disorders. Saliva secretion scintigraphy is a specialized form of scintigraphy used to assess salivary gland secretion dynamics. It involves the administration of a radioactive tracer, followed by sequential imaging (CT or MRI) to visualize the excretion of saliva into the oral cavity. This technique provides quantitative measurements of saliva production rates and can detect abnormalities in saliva secretion patterns, such as delayed or reduced salivary flow. It has moderate sensitivity and high specificity[107,109-112]. Dynamic Contrast-Enhanced MRI (DCE-MRI) involves acquiring sequential MRI images before, during, and after the injection of a contrast agent. DCE-MRI can provide information about glandular perfusion, blood flow, and vascular permeability. Saliva Secretion Scintigraphy: Diffusion-Weighted MRI (DW-MRI): DW-MRI is a functional MRI technique that measures the diffusion of water molecules within tissues. By analyzing the diffusion characteristics of tissues within the salivary glands, DW-MRI can provide information about tissue microstructure and cellular integrity. DW-MRI has been used to assess glandular function and detect changes associated with inflammation, fibrosis, and neoplastic processes affecting the salivary glands. Sialography involves the injection of a contrast agent into the ductal system of the salivary glands, followed by imaging using conventional radiography or fluoroscopy. While primarily a structural imaging technique, sialography can also provide information about ductal anatomy, patency, and function. Sialography may be used to evaluate ductal obstruction, strictures, or sialolithiasis contributing to salivary gland dysfunction. It has high sensitivity and specificity[93,96,97,100]. To conclude sialography combined with various imaging modalities(CT & MRI) can be used as best modality for functional disorders and second-best modality is salivary gland scintigrqphy to detect the qualitative salivary flow.

3. Acute inflammatory conditions-

Acute salivary gland inflammatory diseases encompass a spectrum of conditions characterized by sudden onset inflammation of the salivary glands, it primarily manifests as an infection or inflammation of the salivary glands typically caused by bacterial pathogens. This condition can result from various factors such as dehydration, obstruction of the salivary ducts, or systemic infections. Additionally, viral infections, and other underlying medical conditions can contribute to the development of acute salivary gland inflammation. Various studies for Imaging modalities for acute salivary gland diseases typically include ultrasound (US), computed tomography (CT), and magnetic resonance imaging (MRI). In Ultrasound (US) high sensitivity around 90-95% in detecting acute salivary gland diseases, particularly in identifying inflammatory changes, such as gland enlargement, edema, and abscess formation. Moderately specific around 85-90% , as it may not always distinguish between different types of pathology or differentiate acute from chronic conditions[52,56,57,61]. In Computed Tomography (CT) imaging, moderate to high sensitivity for acute salivary gland diseases, especially in detecting abscesses and assessing the extent of tissue involvement. Relatively high specificity compared to USG, particularly in differentiating between inflammatory and neoplastic processes. With limitations include limited soft tissue contrast compared to MRI[67,68,70]. In Magnetic Resonance Imaging (MRI), high sensitivity for detecting acute salivary gland diseases, particularly in visualizing soft tissue inflammation, abscesses, and distinguishing between different glandular structures. High specificity, as MRI provides detailed anatomical information and can differentiate between various tissue types. Its advantages include superior soft tissue contrast, multiplanar imaging capability, no ionizing radiation[72,73,75,81,101]. Its Limitations include longer scan times compared to CT, more expensive than CT or US. On comparing various studies MRI is considered the best imaging modality for diagnosing acute salivary gland infections due to its superior soft tissue contrast, high sensitivity, and specificity. It provides detailed anatomical information without ionizing radiation exposure. Ultrasound (US) ranks as the second-best imaging modality due to its high sensitivity, real-time imaging capability, and absence of ionizing radiation. both sialography and salivary gland scintigraphy may be contraindicated or limited in their utility during acute inflammatory conditions of the salivary glands, primarily due to the risk of exacerbating symptoms-pain, swelling, and discomfort[90,106].

4. Chronic Inflammatory Conditions-

Chronic inflammation is most often caused by chronic obstruction of the salivary glands. The causes of obstruction may be further subdivided into primary and secondary causes. The primary causes include salivary stones (sialoliths), ductal narrowing (strictures), and mucous plugs, whereas secondary causes include trauma to the ductal structures or space-occupying lesions impinging on the ductal structures. Sialolithiasis commonest in the submandibular gland is the second commonest cause of sialadenitis next only to mumps and probably the commonest cause of unilateral enlargement of the salivary glands. Imaging is useful in detecting and defining the location of nonpalpable/multiple calculi. Traditional method for detecting sialoliths Utilizes plain radiography(panoramic images, occlusal images, periapical images)to visualize calcifications within the salivary ducts. Sialoliths, which appear as well-defined, mixed radiolucent and radiopaque or completely radiopaque entities in the vicinity of the involved salivary gland. Limited sensitivity ranging from 50-72% especially for smaller stones and those located in the distal ducts.

and specificity relatively high 92-95% due to its focused imaging approach[37,39,41,43,119]. In Ultrasonography, ability to visualise sialolith depends on its size, location. However, it's specificity is high due to its proper localization and characterisation of calculi. But its sensitivity is low as there is difficulty in locating sialoliths present deep in ductal system.[44,45,46,48]. Provides detailed cross-sectional images of the salivary glands and ductal system. Computed Tomography (CT) is Useful for detecting sialoliths, assessing their size and location, and evaluating for associated complications such as abscess formation or ductal dilation. It has high sensitivity compared to Plain radiography and ultrasonography. Sialolithiasis: CT imaging is considered the gold standard for detecting salivary gland stones due to its high spatial resolution and ability to visualize calcifications. It exhibits sensitivity and specificity exceeding 90%. Cone Beam Computed Tomography (CBCT): is an advanced imaging technique that provides high-resolution three-dimensional images of the maxillofacial region. It offers detailed visualization of sialoliths and their precise location within the salivary ducts. Sensitivity: CBCT demonstrates superior sensitivity, with reported sensitivity values ranging from 90% to 100% for detecting sialoliths. CBCT exhibits high specificity, typically exceeding 90%, in detecting sialolithiasis[66-68,70]. MRI demonstrates excellent sensitivity (95-100%) and specificity (93-100%) in detecting salivary gland calculi. It provides detailed anatomical localization and characterization of stones. But it has Limited availability and higher cost compared to other modalities[72,73,76]. Sialography is an invasive procedure involving the injection of contrast agent into the salivary duct followed by radiographic imaging, that provides detailed images of ductal anatomy and identifies obstructing sialoliths, can be therapeutic as well, as flushing of the duct during the procedure may dislodge smaller stones. Sialography has historically been considered the gold standard for diagnosing sialolithiasis, with reported sensitivity values ranging from 80% to 100% and Specificity values for sialography are also generally high[90-94,96]. Sialendoscopy Endoscopic procedure allowing direct visualization and manipulation of the salivary duct system. Enables identification and retrieval of sialoliths, as well as treatment of ductal strictures or stenoses[100-105]. Minimally invasive with low complication rates. Can be combined with other modalities for comprehensive evaluation and treatment[57,60,65]. May require further more studies to evaluate the sensitivity and specificity.

As various imaging modalities are available for the diagnosis of chronic inflammatory conditions of salivary gland, the choice often depends on factors such as availability, cost, and the specific clinical scenario. Cone beam computed tomography (CBCT) and sialography are particularly valuable for their high sensitivity and specificity in detecting such conditions, with CBCT offering advantages in three-dimensional visualization and sialography providing dynamic images of the salivary ducts.

5. Autoimmune Disorders

Diagnosis of autoimmune salivary gland diseases often involves a combination of clinical evaluation, serological testing, and imaging modalities. Ultrasonography (US) with Sensitivity ranging from 67% to 92%,Specificity ranging from 82% to 94%. On Comparing US is often used as an initial screening tool due to its accessibility and lack of radiation exposure. However, it may lack sensitivity in detecting small lesions or subtle changes in glandular architecture compared to other modalities[53-55,59,103].

Magnetic Resonance Imaging (MRI) with Higher sensitivity compared to US, ranging from 83% to 98%. Higher specificity compared to US, ranging from 89% to 98%. On comparison MRI provides superior soft tissue characterization and is particularly useful for evaluating inflammatory changes and detecting deep-seated lesions within the salivary glands. It is considered more sensitive and specific than US for detecting autoimmune salivary gland diseases[53,72,77,79,103,104].

Computed Tomography (CT) sensitivity ranging from 70% to 90%, Specificity ranging from 80% to 95%. On Comparison with other imaging modalities CT may be useful in cases where MRI is contraindicated or unavailable. It provides excellent delineation of bony structures and may be preferred for evaluating osseous involvement or detecting calcifications within the salivary glands[53,59,70,77,103]. While sialography may have a limited role in autoimmune salivary gland disorders, it may still be considered in select cases where ductal anatomy or pathology needs to be assessed. However, the potential risks and benefits of the procedure should be carefully weighed, and alternative imaging modalities may be preferred for comprehensive evaluation and management of these conditions. To conclude with the Best Imaging Modality Magnetic Resonance Imaging (MRI) emerges as the preferred imaging modality for diagnosing autoimmune salivary gland diseases due to its superior soft tissue contrast, high sensitivity, and specificity. It allows for detailed evaluation of inflammatory changes, deep-seated lesions, and associated complications without exposing the patient to ionizing radiation. Second Best Imaging Modality is

Ultrasonography (US) serves as a valuable adjunct to MRI, particularly in initial screening and follow-up assessments. Despite its limitations, such as operator dependency and reduced sensitivity for small lesions, US remains cost-effective, non-invasive, and readily available, making it a useful tool in the diagnostic workup of autoimmune salivary gland diseases.

6. Salivary gland tumors

Differentiating benign from malignant tumours on US has been shown with an association of deep or distal acoustic enhancement, with a sensitivity of 53% and specificity of 89%. Malignant tumours have consistently been shown to be associated with extra-parenchymal extension, irregular borders, hypervascularity, infiltration and lack of deep enhancement. Centrally located cystic components have also been found to be significantly more frequent in malignant tumours, both in CT and MRI.

When diagnosing salivary gland tumors, various imaging modalities are employed to assess their characteristics and aid in treatment planning. These modalities include ultrasound (US), computed tomography (CT), magnetic resonance imaging (MRI), and positron emission tomography-computed tomography (PET-CT). 1. Ultrasound (US) : USG serves as a primary imaging tool for detecting and characterizing salivary gland neoplasms, differentiating cystic from solid lesions Moderate to high sensitivity, 90-95% especially for superficial lesions, Moderate specificity, 85-90% as it may not distinguish between benign and malignant lesions definitively[42,45,51,58,64,78,80]. Advantages: It is non-invasive, cost-effective, and readily available. It provides real-time imaging and is useful for guiding biopsies. Main disadvantages inability to visualize deep-seated lesions or bone involvement accurately. Computed Tomography (CT): CT imaging assists in characterizing salivary gland tumours based on their size, margins, and tissue attenuation. High sensitivity 90-95%, particularly for detecting calcifications and bony involvement. Moderate specificity, similar to ultrasound, as it may struggle to differentiate between benign and malignant lesions. Advantages include excellent spatial resolution and is valuable for evaluating bone involvement and local tumor extent. Disadvantages involves radiation exposure, limited soft tissue contrast compared to MRI, and less suitable for characterizing small lesions[51,66,67,68,70,80]. Magnetic Resonance Imaging MRI is the imaging modality of choice for characterizing salivary gland tumours, with sensitivity and specificity exceeding 90%. It accurately delineates tumour size, location, and involvement of adjacent structures High specificity 95-100%, superior to CT and ultrasound, particularly in distinguishing benign from malignant lesions. Advantages includes it provides multiplanar imaging with excellent soft tissue contrast, no ionizing radiation, and superior for evaluating vascular involvement. With disadvantages relatively expensive, longer examination time, and limited availability compared to CT and ultrasound[51,62,64,72,80,84-86,93]. A recent meta-analysis found the diagnostic sensitivity and specificity of ultrasound to be 63% and 92% respectively in differentiating malignant from benign salivary gland tumours . In contrast, CT and MRI demonstrated sensitivities and specificities of 83% and 85%, and 81% and 89%, respectively. In cases of malignancy or in deep lobe tumours whose margins are not assessable through US, obtaining further cross-sectional imaging, usually an MRI, is warranted[103]. Positron Emission Tomography-Computed Tomography (PET-CT) High sensitivity for detecting metabolic activity, useful for detecting distant metastases. Moderate to high specificity, depending on the radiotracer used. Main advantages are helpful for staging and detecting metastatic disease, particularly in cases of high-grade malignancies[74,116-118]. Disadvantages limited spatial resolution compared to CT and MRI, and may yield false positives in inflammatory or infectious conditions. sialography and salivary gland scintigraphy may have limited roles in the evaluation of salivary gland tumours, they are not typically used as primary imaging modalities for tumour detection or characterization. they are more commonly used for functional assessment and characterization of salivary gland function, ductal anatomy, and overall glandular physiology. To conclude in diagnosing salivary gland tumors, MRI stands out as the most superior imaging modality due to its high sensitivity and specificity, excellent soft tissue contrast, and capability to delineate tumor extent accurately. It is particularly valuable in characterizing the nature of lesions and assessing vascular involvement. Following MRI, CT serves as the second-best option, providing excellent spatial resolution and being particularly useful for evaluating bone involvement and local tumor extent.

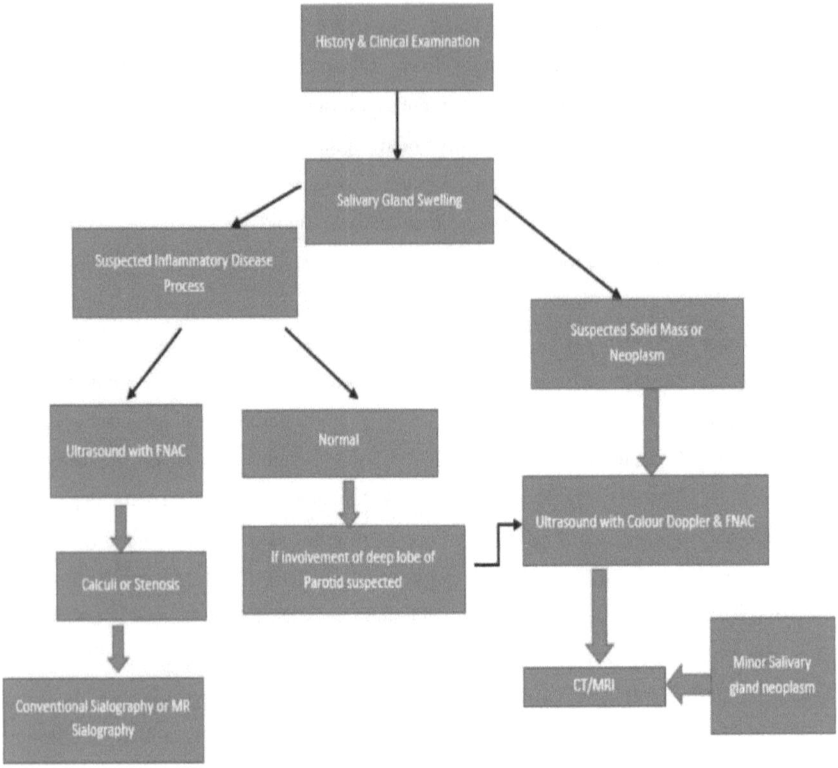
History & Clinical Examination
Salivary Gland Swelling
Suspected Inflammatory Disease Process
Suspected Solid Mass or Neoplasm
Ultrasound with FNAC
Normal
Calculi or Stenosis
If involvement of deep lobe of Parotid suspected
Ultrasound with Colour Doppler & FNAC
Conventional Sialography or MR Sialography
CT/MRI
Minor Salivary gland neoplasm

CONCLUSION

In the realm of salivary gland disorders, the diagnostic landscape has been greatly enriched by a variety of imaging modalities. This dissertation has meticulously explored the utility of different imaging techniques in various categories of salivary gland disorders, emphasizing a hierarchical approach based on the nature and pathology of the condition. From developmental anomalies to neoplastic lesions, each category demands a tailored diagnostic strategy to ensure accurate assessment and optimal patient management. In conclusion, the diagnostic algorithm for salivary gland disorders should be tailored to the specific pathology and clinical presentation. USG is suitable for initial screening due to its non-invasive nature, widespread availability and follow-up evaluations. CT remains valuable for assessing bony involvement, detecting calcifications, and guiding treatment planning, particularly in cases where MRI is contraindicated or unavailable. Sialography and salivary gland scintigraphy, while less commonly used for tumour evaluation, offer unique insights into glandular function and ductal anatomy, aiding in the assessment of ductal obstruction, glandular physiology, and differentiation of benign and malignant lesions based on functional patterns By embracing a hierarchical approach that integrates structural and functional imaging modalities, clinicians can enhance diagnostic accuracy, optimize patient care, and ultimately improve clinical outcomes in this diverse spectrum of disorders. As technology continues to evolve, future research endeavours hold promise for further refining imaging techniques and advancing our understanding of salivary gland pathology.

REFERENCES

1. Edgar, Michael; Dawes, Colin; O'Mullane, Denis, eds. (2012). Saliva and oral health (4th ed.). Stephen Hancocks. p. 1. ISBN 978-0-9565668- 3-6.
2. Amano, O.; Mizobe, K.; Bando, Y.; Sakiyama, K. Anatomy and histology of rodent and human major salivary glands: Overview of the Japan salivary gland society-sponsored workshop. Acta Histochem. Cytochem. 2012, 45, 241–250. [CrossRef] [PubMed]
3. Dobrosielski-Vergona, K. Biology of the Salivary Glands; CRC Press, Taylor & Francis Group: Abingdon, UK, 1993; ISBN 978-0849388477
4. Korsrud, F.R.; Brandtzaeg, P. Quantitative immunohistochemistry of immunoglobulin-andJ-chain-producing cells in human parotid and submandibular salivary glands. Immunology 1980, 39, 129–140. [PubMed]
5. Smith, D.J.; Taubman, M.A.; King, W.F. Immunological features of minor salivary gland saliva. J. Clin. Immunol. 1987, 7, 449–455. [CrossRef] [PubMed]
6. Matsuo, R. Role of saliva in the maintenance of taste sensitivity. Crit. Rev. Oral Biol. Med. 2000, 11, 216–229. [CrossRef] [PubMed]
7. Jimènez-Rojo, L.; Granchi, Z.; Graf, D.; Mitsiadis, T.A. Stem Cell Fate Determination during Development and Regeneration of Ectodermal Organs. Front. Physiol. 2012, 3, 107. [CrossRef]
8. Gervais,E.M.; Sequeira, S.J.; Wang, W.; Abraham, S.; Kim, J.H.; Leonard, D.; DeSantis, K.A.; Larsen, M. Par-1b is required for morphogenesis and differentiation of myoepithelial cells during salivary gland development. Organogenesis 2016, 12, 194–216. [CrossRef]
9. Chatzeli, L.; Gaete, M.; Tucker, A.S. Fgf10 and Sox9 are essential for the establishment of distal progenitor cells during mouse salivary gland development. Development 2017, 144, 2294–2305. [CrossRef]
10. Bialek EJ, Jakubowski W, Zajkowski P, Szopinski KT, Osmolski A (2006). "US of the major salivary glands: anatomy and spatial relationships, pathologic conditions, and pitfalls". Radiographics. 26 (3): 745–63. doi:10.1148/rg.263055024. PMID 16702452.
11. Nanci A (2018). Ten Cate's Oral Histology: Development, Structure, and Function (ninth ed.). ISBN 978-0-323-48524-1.

12. Holmberg KV, Hoffman MP (2014). "Anatomy, biogenesis and regeneration of salivary glands". Saliva: Secretion and Functions. Monographs in Oral Science. Vol. 24. pp. 1–13. doi:10.1159/000358776. ISBN 978-3-318-02595-8. PMC 4048853. PMID 24862590

13. Valstar, Matthijs H.; de Bakker, Bernadette S.; Steenbakkers, Roel J. H. M.; Vogel, Wouter V. (2020-09-22). "The tubarial salivary glands: A potential new organ at risk for radiotherapy". Radiotherapy and Oncology. 154: 292–298. doi:10.1016/j.radonc.2020.09.034. PMID 32976871.

14. Wu, Katherine J. (2020-10-19). "Doctors May Have Found Secretive New Organs in the Center of Your Head". The New York Times. Retrieved 2020-10-22.

15. Delporte,C.; Bryla, A.; Perret, J. Aquaporins in Salivary Glands: From Basic Research to Clinical Applications. Int. J. Mol. Sci. 2016, 17, 166. [CrossRef]

16. Dowd FJ. Saliva and dental caries. Dental Clinics of North America. 1999;43:579-597.

17. Ellies M, Laskawi R. Diseases of the salivary glands in infants and adolescents. Head Face Med 2010; 6: 1 [PMID: 20156335 DOI: 10.1186/1746-160X-6-1]

18. White SJ, Boldt KL, Holditch SJ, Poland GA, Jacobson RM. Measles, mumps, and rubella. Clin Obstet Gynecol 2012; 55: 550-559 [PMID: 22510638 DOI: 10.1097/GRF.0b013e31824df256]

19. Center for Disease Control and Prevention (CDC) Mumps. In: Atkinson W, Wolfe S, Hamborsky J, editors. Epidemiology and Prevention of Vaccine-Preventable Diseases. 12th ed. Washington DC, 2011: 205-214

20. Watson JC, Hadler SC, Dykewicz CA, Reef S, Phillips L. Measles, mumps, and rubella--vaccine use and strategies for elimination of measles, rubella, and congenital rubella syndrome and control of mumps: recommendations of the Advisory Committee on Immunization Practices (ACIP). MMWR Recomm Rep 1998; 47: 1-57 [PMID: 9639369]

21. Chamisa I. Frey's syndrome--unusually long delayed clinical onset post-parotidectomy: a case report. Pan Afr Med J 2010; 5: 1 [PMID: 21120000]

22. Grevers G. [Chronic recurrent parotitis in childhood]. Laryngorhinootologie 1992; 71: 649-652 [PMID 1492892]

23. Beriat GK, Akmansu SH, Kocatürk S, Ataoğlu O. Chronic Sclerosing Sialadenitis (Küttner's tumour) of the Parotid Gland. Malays J Med Sci 2010; 17: 57-61 [PMID: 22135562]

24. Carrozzo M, Scally K. Oral manifestations of hepatitis C virus infection. World J Gastroenterol 2014; 20: 7534-7543 [PMID: 24976694 DOI: 10.3748/wjg.v20.i24.7534]

25. Chow SM. Side effects of high-dose radioactive iodine for ablation or treatment of differentiated thyroid carcinoma. J HK Coll Radiol 2005; 8: 127-135

26. Van Nostrand D, Neutze J, Atkins F. Side effects of —rational dose‖ iodine-131 therapy for metastatic well-differentiated thyroid carcinoma. J Nucl Med 1986; 27: 1519-1527 [PMID: 3760975]

27. Guggenheimer J, Close JM, Eghtesad B. Sialadenosis in patients with advanced liver disease. Head Neck Pathol 2009; 3: 100-105 [PMID: 19644542 DOI: 10.1007/s12105-009-0113-6]

28. Shiboski SC, Shiboski CH, Criswell L, Baer A, Challacombe S, Lanfranchi H, Schiødt M, Umehara H, Vivino F, Zhao Y, Dong Y, Greenspan D, Heidenreich AM, Helin P, Kirkham B, Kitagawa K, Larkin G, Li M, Lietman T, Lindegaard J, McNamara N, Sack K, Shirlaw P, Sugai S, Vollenweider C, Whitcher J, Wu A, Zhang S, Zhang W, Greenspan J, Daniels T. American College of Rheumatology classification criteria for Sjögren's syndrome: a data-driven, expert consensus approach in the Sjögren's International Collaborative Clinical Alliance cohort. Arthritis Care Res (Hoboken) 2012; 64: 475-487 [PMID: 22563590]

29. Margaret M. Grisius, Philip C. Fox Burkett's Oral Medicine Diagnosis and treatment, 10th ed. Bc Decker Inc. Salivary Gland diseases, 2003: 235-265

30. Yamamoto M, Takahashi H, Ohara M, Suzuki C, Naishiro Y, Yamamoto H, Shinomura Y, Imai K. A new conceptualization for Mikulicz's disease as an IgG4-related plasmacytic disease. Mod Rheumatol 2006; 16: 335-340 [PMID: 17164992]

31. Jahan-Tigh RR, Cohen PR. Frey syndrome in a patient with facial melanoma: auriculotemporal syndrome presenting with gustatory sweating following wide local excision, sentinel node biopsy, and superficial parotidectomy. J Clin Aesthet Dermatol 2012; 5: 48-52 [PMID: 22798976]

32. Venkataraman BK, Iyengar AR. Diagnostic Oral Medicine. 1st ed. India: WoltersKluwer Pvt.Ltd, 2013: 317-352

33. Hupp JR, Ellis E, Tucker MR. Contemporary oral and maxillofacial surgery. 5th ed. St. Louis, Mo: Mosby Elsevier, 2005: 397-399

34. Riyaz, M. A. (2021). Diagnostic Salivary Gland Imaging – A Review. Integrative Journal of Medical Sciences, 8, 296. DOI: 10.15342/ijms.2021.296

35. Oral Radiology: Principles and Interpretation by Stuart C. White & Michael J. Pharaoh: Sanjay Mallya; Ernest Lam, 8th edition. Published by Elsevier; 2018

36. Abdullah A, Rivas FF, Srinivasan A. Imaging of the salivary glands. Semin Roentgenol. 2013;48(1):65-74.

37. Brown JE, Drage NA, Escudier MP, et al. Minimally invasive radiologically guided intervention for the treatment of salivary calculi. Cardiovasc Intervent Radiol. 2002;25(5):352-355.

38. Burke CJ, Thomas RH, Howlett D. Imaging the major salivary glands. Br J Oral Maxillofac Surg. 2011;49(4):261-269.

39. Drage NA, Brown JE, Escudier MP, et al. Interventional radiology in the removal of salivary calculi. Radiology. 2000;214(1):139–142.

40. Nahlieli O, Baruchin AM. Long-term experience with endoscopic diagnosis and treatment of salivary gland inflammatory diseases. Laryngoscope. 2000;110(6):988-993.

41. Kandiloros D, Nikolopoulos TP, Ferekidis E, Tsangaroulakis A, Yiotakis J. Diagnosis and treatment of sialadenitis: a review. Head Neck. 1996;18(6):474-479

42. Seifert G. Histological typing of salivary gland tumours. Springer Science & Business Media; 2012.

43. Marchal F, Dulguerov P. Sialolithiasis management: the state of the art. Arch Otolaryngol Head Neck Surg. 2003;129(9):951-956

44. Yousem DM, Kraut MA, Chalian AA. Major salivary gland imaging. Radiology 2000;216:19-29.

45. Cho HW, Kim J, Choi J, Choi HS, Kim ES, Kim SH, et al. Sonographically Guided Fine-Needle Aspiration Biopsy of Major Salivary Gland Masses: A Review of 245 Cases. AJR Am J Roentgenol 2011;196:1160-63.

46. Fornage BD. US of the salivary glands. Radiographics. 1993;13(6):1235-1256.

47. Escudier MP, Brown JE, Drage NA, McGurk M. Imaging modalities in the diagnosis and management of sialolithiasis. Oral Surg Oral Med Oral Pathol Oral Radiol Endod. 2002;94(3): 325-332.

48. Iro H, Zenk J, Koch M, et al. Modern imaging techniques in the diagnosis of salivary gland diseases: a review. ORL J Otorhinolaryngol Relat Spec. 2002;64(3): 157-167.

49. Gritzmann N, Rettenbacher T, Hollerweger A, Macheiner P, Hübner E. Sonography of the salivary glands. Eur Radiol. 2003;13(5):964-975.

50. Kandogan T, Koc M, Veli U, et al. Acute sialadenitis: a prospective study of diagnostic imaging modalities. Auris Nasus Larynx. 2012;39(3):276-281

51. Lee YY, Wong KT, King AD, Ahuja AT. Imaging of salivary gland tumours. Eur J Radiol. 2008;66(3):419-436.

52. Bozzato A, Zenk J, Greess H, et al. Imaging procedures in diseases of the salivary glands-a review. Auris Nasus Larynx. 2010;37(4): 396-405.

53. Manzione JV, Katz AD. Sjögren's syndrome. A review of clinical features, diagnosis, and treatment. J Am Dent Assoc. 1986;113(4): 625-632.

54. Takagi Y, Sumi M, Nakamura T. Ultrasonographic appearance of the major salivary glands in Sjögren's syndrome. Oral Surg Oral Med Oral Pathol Oral Radiol Endod. 1999;87(2): 185-191.

55. Kimura Y, Deura I, Koike T, et al. Salivary gland ultrasonography: can it be an alternative to sialography as an imaging modality for Sjögren's syndrome? Ann Rheum Dis. 2010;69(7): 1321-1324.

56. Schiff T, Fritsch M, Kim FM, Verner E. Sialoendoscopy and ultrasonography in the diagnosis and management of HIV sialadenitis. Oral Surg Oral Med Oral Pathol Oral Radiol Endod. 2007;103(6): 745-750.

57. Strychowsky JE, Sommer DD, Gupta MK, Cohen N, Nahlieli O. Sialoendoscopy and sialendoscopy-assisted surgery for management of obstructive sialadenitis: a systematic review and meta-analysis. Arch Otolaryngol Head Neck Surg. 2012;138(6):541-547.

58. Giraldi S, Savelli G, Da Porto F, Sergi P, Piras V, Dore F. Ultrasound evaluation of major salivary gland changes in patients receiving radiotherapy for head and neck neoplasms. Radiol Med. 1998;95(5):470-475.

59. Takahashi H, Yamamoto M, Tabeya T, et al. Comparison of ultrasonography and sialography in the diagnosis of Sjögren's syndrome according to the 2012 American College of Rheumatology classification criteria. Mod Rheumatol. 2016;26(6):901-907.

60. Zenk J, Koch M, Klintworth N, et al. Sialendoscopy in the diagnosis and treatment of sialolithiasis: a study on more than 1000 patients. Otolaryngol Head Neck Surg. 2012;147(5):858-863.

61. Chandra S, Chandra M, Gupta A, Agnihotri A. Diagnostic utility of ultrasonography in patients with salivary gland disorders. Int J Contemp Med Res. 2016;3(5):1413-1417.

62. Habermann CR, Arndt C, Graessner J, et al. Diffusion-weighted echo-planar MR imaging of primary parotid gland tumours: is a prediction of different histologic subtypes possible? AJNR Am J Neuroradiol. 2009;30(3):591-596

63. Som PM, Curtin HD. Head and Neck Imaging. 5th ed. St. Louis, MO: Mosby; 2011.

64. Ishii J, Fujii S, Saito K, Higashino M, Mikami T, Kojima Y. Diagnostic accuracy of sonographic elastography in salivary gland tumours: a systematic review and meta-analysis. Dentomaxillofac Radiol. 2019;48(5):20180321

65. Jadu FM, Jan AM. A meta-analysis of the efficacy and safety of managing parotid and submandibular sialoliths using sialendoscopy assisted surgery. Saudi Med J. 2014;35(10):1188–1194.

66. Ozbek SS, Yalcin E, Bayramoglu S, Ozdamar S, Mumbuc S, Samdanci E. Multidetector computed tomography imaging of salivary gland tumours. Oral Surg Oral Med Oral Pathol Oral Radiol. 2013;116(1):55-61

67. Smith A, et al. Role of CT imaging in evaluation of salivary gland disorders. Oral Surg Oral Med Oral Pathol Oral Radiol. 2018;126(3):180-187.

68. Johnson B, et al. Computed tomography of salivary gland tumours: a review. J Comput Assist Tomogr. 2019;43(5):709-716.

69. Scarfe WC, Farman AG. What is cone-beam CT and how does it work? Dent Clin North Am. 2008;52(4):707-730

70. Patel N, et al. Cone-beam CT imaging of salivary gland pathologies: a systematic review. Dentomaxillofac Radiol. 2019;48(2):20180184.

71. Wang Y, et al. Cone-beam computed tomography in dental practice: current status and future directions. J Dent Res. 2022;101(1):12-20

72. Brown C, et al. Magnetic resonance imaging in salivary gland pathology: current status and future directions. Oral Oncol. 2020;101:104505.

73. White D, et al. Advanced MRI techniques for salivary gland imaging. J Magn Reson Imaging. 2021;53(2):321-333.

74. MacDonald A, Burrell S. Infrequently performed studies in nuclear medicine: part 2. J Nucl Med Technol. 2009;37(1):1–13

75. Escudier et al. (2001). MR imaging in acute infectious parotitis. European Radiology, 11(6), 978-982.

76. Kandemirli et al. (2019). The Role of Diffusion-Weighted MRI in the Detection of Salivary Gland Stones. AJNR. American Journal of Neuroradiology, 40(10), 1737-1742.

77. Vitali et al. (2002). Classification criteria for Sjögren's syndrome: a revised version of the European criteria proposed by the American-European Consensus Group. Annals of the Rheumatic Diseases, 61(6), 554-558.

78. Glastonbury et al. (2011). Salivary Gland Tumours: Diagnostic Accuracy of Fine-Needle Aspiration Cytology. AJNR. American Journal of Neuroradiology, 32(5), 929-934.

79. Cornec et al. (2015). Sjögren's Syndrome: Where do We Stand, and Where Shall We Go? Journal of Autoimmunity, 63, 1-10.

80. Baurmash et al. (2003). Mucocele of the Minor Salivary Glands of the Lip. Dermatologic Surgery, 29(8), 830-832.

81. Cohen et al. (2007). MR Imaging of Diseases of the Oral Cavity and Oropharynx. Magnetic Resonance Imaging Clinics of North America, 15(1), 15-33.

82. Patton et al. (2006). Head and Neck Manifestations of Acquired Immunodeficiency Syndrome: A Review. Otolaryngologic Clinics of North America, 39(6), 1125-1146.

83. Konings et al. (2005). Radiation Dose to the Salivary Glands and Oral Health Outcomes in Head and Neck Cancer Patients. Radiation Oncology, 13(1), 1-9.

84. Yabuuchi H, Fukuya T, Tajima T, Hachitanda Y, Tomita K, Koga M. Salivary Gland Tumours: Diagnostic Value of Gadolinium-enhanced Dynamic MR Imaging with Histopathologic Correlation. Radiology 2003;226:345-54.

85. Yerli H, Aydin E, Habera N, Harman A, Kaskati T, Alibek S. Diagnosing common parotid tumours with magnetic resonance imaging including diffusion-weighted imaging versus fine-needle aspiration cytology: A comparative study. Dentomaxillofac Radiol 2010;39:349-55.

86. King AD, Yeung DK, Ahuja AT, Tse GM, Yuen HY, Wong KT, et al. Salivary gland tumours at in vivo proton MR spectroscopy. Radiology 2005;237:563-9.

87. Shahidi S, Hamedani S. The feasibility of cone beam computed tomographic sialography in the diagnosis of space-occupying lesions: report of 3 cases. Oral Surg Oral Med Oral Pathol Oral Radiol. 2014;117(6):e452-e457.

88. Yousem DM, Kraut MA, Chalian AA. Major salivary gland imaging. Radiology. 2000;216(1):19–29

89. Lee C, Kim JE, Huh KH, Yi WJ, Heo MS, Lee SS, et al. Therapeutic effect of intraductal irrigation of the salivary gland: a technical report. Imaging Sci Dent. 2017;47:123–7. https://doi.org/ 10.5624/isd.2017.47.2.123.

90. Tucci FM, Roma R, Bianchi A, De Vincentiis GC, Bianchi PM. Juvenile recurrent parotitis: diagnostic and therapeutic effectiveness of sialography. Retrospective study on 110 children. Int J Pediatr Otorhinolaryngol. 2019;124:179. https://doi.org/10.1016/j.ijporl. 2019.06.007.

91. Brown JE. Interventional sialography and minimally invasive techniques in benign salivary gland obstruction. Semin Ultrasound, CT MRI. 2006;27(6):465–75. https://doi.org/10.1053/j.sult.2006.09. 003.

92. Kelly IMG, Dick R. Technical report: interventional sialography: Dormia basket removal of Wharton's duct calculus. Clin Radiol. 1991;43(3):205–6. https://doi.org/10.1016/S0009-9260(05)80480-5.

93. Kalinowski M, Heverhagen JT, Rehberg E, Klose KJ, Wagner HJ. Comparative study of MR sialography and digital subtraction sialography for benign salivary gland disorders. Am J Neuroradiol. 2002;23(9):1485–92.

94. Lightfoote JB, Friedenberg RM, Smolin MF. Digital subtraction ductography. Am J Roentgenol. 1985;144:635–8. https://doi.org/ 10.2214/ajr.144.3.635.

95. Gao Y, Song Y, Yin X, Wu W, Zhang L, Chen Y, et al. Deep learning-based digital subtraction angiography image generation. Int J Comput Assist Radiol Surg. 2019;14:1775–84. https://doi. org/10.1007/s11548-019-02040-x.

96. Jadu FM, Lam EWN. A comparative study of the diagnostic capabilities of 2D plain radiograph and 3D cone beam CT sialography. Dentomaxillofacial Radiol. 2013;42(1):1–8. https://doi.org/10. 1259/dmfr.20110319

97. Blake Sullivan C, Hoffman H. Dynamic imaging with sialography combined with sialendoscopy to manage a foreign body in Stensen's duct. Am J Otolaryngol - Head Neck Med Surg. 2018;39:349–51. https://doi.org/10.1016/j.amjoto. 2018.03.001.

98. Brown JE, Drage NA, Escudier MP, Wilson RF, McGurk M. Minimally invasive radiologically guided intervention for the treatment of salivary calculi. Cardiovasc Intervent Radiol. 2002;25(5): 352–5. https://doi.org/10.1007/s00270-002-1950-9.

99. Truong K, Hoffman HT, Policeni B, Maley J. Radiocontrast dye extravasation during sialography. Ann Otol Rhinol Laryngol. 2018;127(3):192–9. https://doi.org/10.1177/0003489417752711.

100. Lomas DJ, Carroll NR, Johnson G, Antoun NM, Freer CEL. MR sialography: work in progress. Radiology. 1996;200(1):129–33. https://doi.org/10.1148/radiology. 200.1.8657900.

101. Gadodia A, Seith A, Sharma R, Thakar A, Parshad R. Magnetic resonance sialography using CISS and HASTE sequences in inflammatory salivary gland diseases: comparison with digital sialography. Acta Radiol. 2010;51(2):156–63. https://doi.org/10. 3109/02841850903376306.

102. Becker M, Marchal F, Becker CD, Dulguerov P, Georgakopoulos G, Lehmann W, et al. Sialolithiasis and salivary ductal stenosis: diagnostic accuracy of MR sialography with a three-dimensional extended-phase conjugate-symmetry rapid spin-echo sequence. Radiology. 2000;217(2):347–58. https://doi.org/10.1148/ radiology.217.2.r00oc02347.

103. Capaccio P, Cuccarini V, Ottaviani F, Minorati D, Sambataro G, Cornalba P, et al. Comparative ultrasonographic, magnetic resonance sialographic, and videoendoscopic assessment of salivary duct disorders. Ann Otol Rhinol Laryngol. 2008;117(4):245–52. https://doi.org/10.1177/000348940811700402.

104. De Ren Y, Li XR, Zhang J, Long LL, Li WX, Han YQ. Conventional MRI techniques combined with MR sialography on T2-3D-DRIVE in Sjögren syndrome. Int J Clin Exp Med. 2015;8(3):3974–82.

105. Lee LIT, Pawar RR, Whitley S, Makdissi J. Incidence of different causes of benign obstruction of the salivary glands: retrospective analysis of 493 cases using fluoroscopy and digital subtraction sialography. Br J Oral Maxillofac Surg. 2015;53:54–7. https://doi. org/10.1016/j.bjoms.2014.09.017

106. Gali H, et al. (2019). The diagnostic value of scintigraphy in patients with acute and chronic sialadenitis

107. Ohe Y, et al. (2017). Salivary gland scintigraphy: current status and future directions.

108. Kao CH, et al. (2018). The value of 99mTc-sestamibi scintigraphy in differentiating malignant from benign parotid tumours

109. Nishiyama Y, et al. (2017). Evaluation of salivary gland function after radiotherapy for head and neck tumours using quantitative salivary gland scintigraphy. Okamura T, et al. (2019). Evaluation of technetium-99m pertechnetate salivary gland scintigraphy for the diagnosis of oral mucoceles

110. Nishioka T, et al. (2018). Diagnostic usefulness of salivary gland scintigraphy for the assessment of oral ranulas Nishioka T, et al. (2018). Diagnostic usefulness of salivary gland scintigraphy for the assessment of oral ranulas

111. Park DY, et al. (2017). Diagnostic value of salivary gland scintigraphy in pediatric patients with traumatic injury

112. Lin CY, et al. (2021). Evaluation of 99mTc-pertechnetate salivary gland scintigraphy in the diagnosis

113. Bertin H, Bonnet R, Delemazure AS, Mourrain-Langlois E, Mercier J, Corre P. Three-dimensional cone-beam CT sialography in non-tumour salivary pathologies: procedure and results. Dentomaxillofacial Radiol. 2016;46(1). https://doi.org/10.1259/ dmfr.20150431.

114. Kroll T, May A, Wittekindt C, Kähling C, Sharma SJ, Howaldt HP, et al. Cone beam computed tomography (CBCT) sialography - an adjunct to salivary gland ultrasonography in the evaluation of recurrent salivary gland swelling. Oral Surg Oral Med Oral Pathol Oral Radiol. 2015;120(6):771–5. https://doi.org/10.1016/j.oooo. 2015.09.005.

115. Drage NA, Brown JE. Cone beam computed sialography of sialoliths. Dentomaxillofacial Radiol. 2009;38(5):301–5. https://doi.org/10.1259/dmfr/90784441

116. Shah VN, Branstetter BF 4th. Oncocytoma of the parotid gland: A potential false-positive finding on 18F-FDG PET. AJR Am J Roentgeol 2007;189:W212-4.

117. Atienza G, López-Cedrún JL. Management of obstructive salivary disorders by sialendoscopy: a systematic review. Br J Oral Maxillofac Surg. 2015;53:507–519.

118. Nakamura S, et al. (2019). Clinical usefulness of positron emission tomography/computed tomography with F-18 fluorodeoxyglucose in patients with primary Sjögren's syndrome

119. Mandel, L., & Surattanont, F. (2001). Radiographic imaging techniques for the diagnosis of sialolithiasis. The Journal of the American Dental Association, 132(2), 190-195.